NATURAL FACELIFT

NATURAL FACELIFT

Juliette Kando

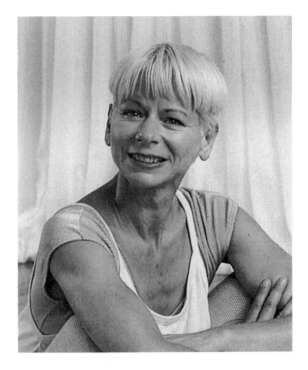

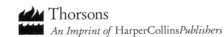
Thorsons
An Imprint of HarperCollins*Publishers*

Thorsons
An Imprint of HarperCollins*Publishers*
77–85 Fulham Palace Road,
Hammersmith, London W6 8JB

Originally published as *The Natural Face Book* 1991
This edition 1998
10 9 8 7 6 5 4 3

© Juliette Kando 1991

Juliette Kando asserts the moral right to
be identified as the author of this work

A catalogue record for this book
is available from the British Library

ISBN 0 7225 3679 8

Printed and bound in Great Britain by
Scotprint Ltd, Musselburgh, Edinburgh

CONTENTS

ACKNOWLEDGEMENTS

I must firstly thank my three children, Miko, Tomi and Kirsty, for teaching me about human movement development from birth onwards and for being respectful and positively critical of my work. I am most grateful to my husband Iain Adam who has taught me proper English and has had to put up with my sneaking into his office at all possible times to use the computer. I wish to thank my friend Tamar Karet who encouraged me to develop my ideas and put them down on paper. This book could not have been written without my work with the late Rudolph Benesh who, through his invention — choreology — opened my eyes to the marvels of movement. Much valuable knowledge comes from Wiet Palar, my Indonesian Yoga teacher and 'Guru' who taught me to listen to my body and harmonize with the surroundings. I will never cease learning from Professor Thomas M. Kando Ph.D., my brother in Sacramento, California who has always forced me to back up hypotheses and utopia with fact. I owe to my twin sister Madeleine Kando MA, D.Th., Dance and Movement Therapist at the Children's Arts corner in Boston, Mass., the discovery that art and health are one. Much inspiration has come from Anna d'Edam and Ed van der Elsken, a unique Dutch photographer couple who have added much style and common sense to my outlook on life. I am greatly indebted to all my friends and clients who, especially in the beginning, served as guinea pigs in the evolution of the facial exercise programme as it is printed here. I want to thank Tina Robinson our beautiful model who has, within a very short period of time, learned to perform the exercises well enough to pose for the illustrations in the book. Lastly and most dearly I want to thank my mother, photographer Ata Kando who, through her work in the Amazonian jungle as far back as the early sixties, has taught me that 'primitive' cultures have a lot to teach us about nature if we want to be a part of it.

Juliette Kando

INTRODUCTION

Development of the System

The system of exercises in this book has grown up out of my own career and interests. After some years as a ballet dancer with the Dutch National Ballet and the Berlin Opera Ballet Company, I worked as a company choreologist for a number of years, putting on large-scale ballet productions in theatres all over the world. But by then I had become a mother of three, and working away from home was no longer what I wanted. In 1982, while on a job in New York, I noticed that on Broadway, there were dance and exercise studios on almost every block, neatly tucked away on the first and second floors, above shops and restaurants. It occurred to me that I could open a similar studio in Kilburn, a fairly rough inner city area in London, where I live with my growing family. The population of Kilburn, like many other inner London areas, comprises people from many different backgrounds, races, ages and states of fitness. Teaching ballet to this very mixed community felt like a great challenge. I had already been teaching ballet to amateurs in central London, but this involved long Tube journeys, high studio rentals and, worst of all a loose, irregular clientele, which is very unrewarding for a teacher. I wanted a studio where ordinary people could come without the intimidation of a semi-professional, competitive, hustling atmosphere so typical of the city centre studios. If we had such a studio, like those on Broadway, in every high street in the country, maybe the British would also gain in vitality, which they lacked so much in comparison to Americans.

So I decided to quit the glamorous life of theatre, and when I had found a suitable building, I founded the Every Body Dance Studios, situated in Kilburn, five minutes from my home. It was a drastic change for me. In the theatre, I had to concentrate on getting large groups of professional dancers to execute set choreographic movements. The job of a choreologist entails teaching dancers the technique and performance of dance movements, musicality and all the other things written in a full choreographic score that make a performance work. Teaching amateurs is a different kettle of fish altogether, but it was a real challenge to teach ordinary, untrained people because it involves educating them to use their bodies in more efficient ways. For example, when people suffer from stiff backs, short hamstrings and so on, the classes are geared towards stretching and bending.

In this situation, dance can become movement and exercise; its function changes from being an expensive art form for the rich to a vital healing practice for "every body". By exploring human movement from its roots, through my own and other people's growing children, by studying other movement disciplines, such as yoga, and also by observing how elderly people coped with the decreasing suppleness in their bodies, a link could be made between the physical shortcomings of ordinary, untrained people and the pure aesthetics of classical ballet. The whole idea behind Every Body was therefore to educate people of all ages to understand their bodies better, as well as other people's bodies.

Since the studio opened, over 2000 regular members of all age groups have benefited from our work at Every Body. One day at the end of a stretch class, when my clients were relaxing to soft music, I caught my own face in the studio mirror and noticed a deeply engraved frown on my forehead. Centrally placed above the eyebrows was another line, short but deep. Together, these two features made me look angry and worried. I looked down to the faces of my clients who were lying on the studio floor. Even the middle-aged to elderly clients looked happy, satisfied and beautifully smooth and wrinkle-free. I looked in the mirror again and wondered why I was looking worried and angry. As soon as the class got up, I noticed that some of their faces too, now showed decades of gravity pulling down on the flesh.

After class when we all met for a snack in the health bar, the lighting was even more unfavourable and I could see that while some of my clients' bodies and postures could easily compete with those of 18-year-olds, their faces had, somewhere along the line, been left behind. Jaw lines were broken by downward-hanging cheek bags, necks were covered in lines and some eyes were drooping down like those of bulldogs. It seemed a shame that the best parts of our well-exercised bodies were covered in clothes. It was then that I realized that something major was missing from the timetable. We were catering for almost every type of movement, people were getting happier and fitter, but the problem of ageing in the face was not being dealt with at all. In fact, my clients often looked better and younger in leotards, when you could see their fit bodies, than they did in street clothes. It occurred to me that if it is possible to tone up a sagging stomach, then surely, it shouldn't be too difficult to tone up a sagging cheek. In the rest of the body, regular use of muscle contraction eliminates fat tissue and firms up muscle tissue. Co-ordination (the conscious use of particular muscle groups to move particular areas) must be the basis for any muscular development in the body as well as in the face.

Later, while walking home, I tried to perform a "cheek contraction" and I noticed to my dismay that I was blinking an eye instead. I concluded that this inadequacy of performance was as clumsy as a baby trying to feed itself in terms of localized co-ordination control. I instantly declared myself facially crippled and embarked upon developing the facial exercises which later became this book.

In the beginning, I exercised in secret, in the closed bathroom, as I wasn't at all sure if it would work. As soon as I started exercising chin ups, cheek contractions, eyebrow raisers and so on, people began to compliment me on my looks for my age and started asking me how to get rid of a double chin, or eye bags. I have always had to be my own best advertisement in my work, so before I could answer those questions, I had to find out how to resolve them for myself. Now that I knew a little more about the face, I was able to give specific exercises to people with specific problems and they worked.

In most cases, it appeared, someone's face could be corrected with specifically directed exercises in the same way that any "body" was taught to behave, namely, to be symmetrically well-balanced, supple, strong and co-ordinated. By developing selected exercise programmes for each individual, great changes can take place, even in an ageing face.

Principles of the Exercises

Isometrics and callisthenics are trendy words for exercise of one kind or another and their meaning is briefly explained here, just in case you wondered what they were.

Isometrics

Isometrics describes repetitious exercises of equal measure. The term is often incorrectly used by teachers to describe minimal movement or isolation of small muscle units to tone a particular area. Although you will be doing exercises of a repetitive nature, they are not isometric but, as you will see, most exercises are based on an initial increase in power, a hold and finally a decrease in power. The term isometrics is too specific and not used in this book. Isolation of muscle units and minimal movements are explained in Chapter 3, Method, Assessment and Course Charts.

Callisthenics

Callisthenics describes exercises to achieve bodily health and grace of movement. The term comes from the Greek *kallos* — beauty — and *sthenos* — strength. The term callisthenics is often used in error by teachers to describe movement against resistance. The whole essence of this book is callisthenic — in other words, you will indeed achieve bodily health and grace if you work through the exercises conscientiously. Movement against some form of resistance is often used in the exercises and its technique is clearly explained in each case. The term callisthenics is too general in the wide context of the facial exercises and so will not be used in the book.

The principles in this book come from a wide variety of disciplines covering ballet, yoga, massage, acupressure, herbalism, aromatherapy, and choreology — all of which are really just specialist terms for basic human faculties like taste, feel, touch, smell, rhythm, movement and dynamics. The principles used here are not "new" or trendy. Most of them have been tried and tested over thousands of years. Only choreology and the amalgamation of principles taken from such wide sources are new and unique to my face rejuvenation system. Below are short descriptions of how each discipline fits into the overall plan.

Ballet

If the training method of ballet can make a body supple, slender and expressive, I reasoned, then some of its principles could also apply to the face. The development of the facial exercise programme is based in part on line, design, symmetry, rhythm and balance — all balletic attributes.

Yoga

The ancient discipline of yoga teaches that the body and the mind (the self) are one. Yoga uses breathing as a connection between the self and the external world in its practice to maintain the body in top form. Yogic principles are a great help for concentration and breathing while doing the facial exercises.

Massage

Massage is just another form of movement: in this case, the body moves passively, it is moved by someone else. A rocking boat or fast-moving train gives the body some form of massage. Passive movement allows bits of the body to be moved by an external force rather than muscular action. Inactive movement of body parts and breathing techniques allow free flow of energy, life force, prana, chi, — this thing that exists in every language but has never been put on a microscope slide. It cannot be cut out of the body and dissected, but it can be felt as energy flowing through your lungs, nostrils, nerves, muscles and bones, right down into your toenails.

When massage is well applied, it will release tension in any part of the body, but that is not all it can do for you. As the paths of energy are cleaned of blockages and muscular spasm, the way is cleared for regeneration and health to move freely through the body. This is why movement is so crucial to health. Passive movement is the most regenerating type, which is lucky, because it means you won't get tired at all! On the contrary, the exercises in this book are going to give you a real uplift in face and soul alike. Three different massage techniques are used in the book, and are dealt with in Chapter 4.

Acupressure

Acupressure is manual pressure applied to a specific slightly depressed point on the body which is known in Chinese medicine to mark channels of energy (meridians). For example, the stomach meridian starts at the lower part of the eye socket and goes down as far as the second toe. These meridians, again, cannot be seen when a body is cut open but they can be explained through movement. There are books with diagrams of meridians but you can also find them by experimenting with your own body. For example, to feel the very long bladder meridian, sit on the floor with the legs straight and feet together. Now bend forwards and let your body relax. If you have difficulty sitting like this, prop up your back against a wall. (If you are sitting on a chair reading this book, get off it and go and sit on the floor!) Now to feel the connection between your left foot and your head, flex your left foot and bend your head down further. You are feeling a strong pulling sensation all the way down the back of your left leg, your spine and neck. It is as if someone had tied an elastic band to your second left toe, wrapped it around the back of the left leg, the spine and tied the other end to your skull. This band represents a meridian.

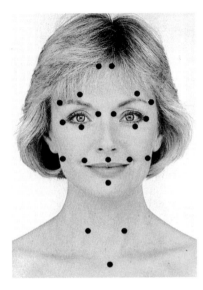

Fig 1: The facial acupressure map

Along its path are several points. Regard the meridians as lines on a railway map, with the acupressure points as the stations. Along the bladder meridian are several points at the back of the ankle, knee, under the hip joint, along the vertebral column and neck to terminate at the inner eye corner. If there is a blockage somewhere along the meridian, it is often enough to unblock one point to release the cause of trouble, which may be in quite a different place from the pressure point. For example if someone has a terrible pain in their lower back, thinking it might be kidney trouble, it may turn out that with relaxation, massage and acupressure the pain goes away. The pain was probably caused by sitting in an unbalanced position for too long, creating muscle spasm which blocked a vital meridian. If the position is resumed, the pain will return, otherwise it will stay away. In this way acupressure is used to release tension spots in the shoulders and neck and to erase wrinkles in the face. Fig 1 gives the main acupressure points in the face and these are referred to in certain exercises given later.

Herbalism and Aromatherapy

Long ago, people discovered how to extract the essential scent from a plant by catching its concentrated oil through a vaporizing device. The Chinese knew thousands of years ago that etheric oils prepared from certain herbs, fruit and flowers had strong healing and cosmetic powers. The knowledge spread to India, Persia and especially Egypt. Medicine in old Egypt was largely based on the use of aromatic substances, and the strong disinfecting properties of the scents were used in the mummification process. The oils have the same healing properties as the plants they are made from, and they are much stronger. Because they are so concentrated (it takes 30 roses to make one drop of rose oil) you only need a few drops of essential oil in any preparation. Chapter 4 sets out in detail how you can prepare individualized natural cosmetic products to clean, massage and feed your face.

Choreology

The research I have carried out for this book has all been annotated in movement notation (choreology). Choreology was invented in London in 1955 by Rudolph Benesh. Benesh was an accountant by profession; music and painting were his hobbies. His wife, who was a ballet dancer, asked him to invent a system for annotating dance steps. Rudolph Benesh was not a mover himself. He was a small, shy, bearded man who did most of the research and development on his notation system sitting down at a desk. The signs and symbols he developed to describe movement down to the minutest detail had to be foolproof. If someone who had just come in could read an unseen movement that someone else had written in his sign language, he was satisfied.

I worked for many years with Benesh in the latter stages of the completion of his system. The language Rudolph Benesh developed is a purely kinetic language, directly related to visible moves and positions, and detached from any kind of verbal description. The advantage of using a specifically-designed annotation system for movement is that it describes movement itself rather than an anatomical, functional, scientific or poetic verbal translation of movement. It gives the observer an insight into the nature of movement, its laws and limitations and also its great potential for enhancing life.

Rudolph Benesh gave choreology the following definition: the scientific and aesthetic study of movement.It is nowadays widely used in choreography, physiotherapy, anthropology and ergonomics. Choreology has provided invaluable data throughout the research stages of this book, which could not have been written without it. Although the exercise programme is derived from data retrieved choreologically, you don't have to have any specialized knowledge of choreology to execute the movements in the book, as I have given you full instructions.

Benefits of Using the System

The benefits gained from doing the exercises in this book are twofold. You will become healthier and more beautiful all at once. Really good health in mind and body is synonymous with happiness, and together they reflect beauty. So whereas your initial interest in the subject was, (like my own, at first) vanity, the whole process soon turns into something else. Losing ugly double chins, eye bags and wrinkles makes you beautiful, but who had ever thought that it would make you happy and healthy as well?

On reflection, this cannot be otherwise. What we really dislike about a double chin or puffy eyes is not their appearance, but what causes their appearance to emerge in the first place, namely, a stiff neck and stuffed-up blocked sinuses. We may not be aware of this, but nevertheless, the negativity of ugliness is not unfounded. Ugliness stems from minor illness factors somewhere inside the body. In addition to looking better, you will begin to see, hear, taste, eat, speak, sing and express yourself better as well. In fact, anything the face does will improve. Ageing will become a pleasant and exciting time instead of the beginning of the humiliating rejection so many senior citizens experience today.

It doesn't matter if you are 25 or 75. Working through the exercises given in this book will give anyone a new boost of life which will last for ever. The younger you start the better, but age is immaterial: the face can recover from abuse or lack of vitality at any age. So it is never too late to start.

Facial Connections, Self-image and Confidence

Unlike other books on beauty which treat the face like an isolated mask, I soon found out that working on the face entails working on the whole self as it is impossible to detach one from the other. For each client, treatment of a facial problem began by looking at the whole person. So we have to start with posture, balance and carriage of movements. This is dealt with in Chapter 1 which is, in part, written for all my clients who used to have so little confidence in themselves that at first they really hated their features and bodies. Chapter 1, which deals with your self-image, works systematically through the whole skeleton, starting at the feet, to give you a strong, balanced stance and posture in preparation for the more detailed exercises on the head and face. Correct postural alignment is vital to neck, shoulder and head carriage. It is important to know the exercises for good posture and movement habits before attempting to work on the face, or the facial exercises won't be as effective. (It's no use trying to hang a beautiful painting on a decaying wall).

The rest of the book deals mainly with facial exercises and how to choose your own self-programmed course of exercises, to assess improvement in your face and to progressively change your choice of exercises to suit your own needs. You will also see how the face is linked to the scalp and the rest of the body.

What Does it Involve and How Much Time Will it Take?

You should spend 10 minutes daily for two weeks as an introductory course, following all the instructions in sequence. After the first fortnight, rest for a week. Don't be impatient and carry on after the second week: the break is part of the course design. Your body needs that time to allow all the new instructions to settle in and to condition itself to losing some bad habits before it is ready to take in any more new programming. After this week's break you are asked to spend 10 minutes only every other day learning one or two new exercises each time, with a monthly 30-minute booster programme. After one month, you are asked to go back to Chapter 3 and make a new assessment chart to modify your course to a more advanced stage. The exercises are marked according to their level of difficulty: beginners, intermediate or advanced. You don't have to learn all the exercises, there are far too many for that. But once a month you should make a new assessment chart and choose progressively harder exercises for your problems. If you are not sure which exercises you should choose, start with the beginners' level, then when they become easy to do, move onto a higher level. There will be many advanced exercises that you won't be able to do at first, so just keep them for a later stage. You will get to them in good time.

After a fortnight, your facial movement patterns will already be more co-ordinated, conscious and efficient. Efficiency is time saving. You will be practising while doing other everyday things like brushing your teeth or putting on your make-up, or even in the bath, or when eating dinner, by controlling habits.

After about the third month, the exercises should have become part of your daily routine for ever and you should have no more need for the book except, I hope, to show it to your friends, and as a source of reference for emergencies: for example, if when you have an important interview but have just woken up with a hangover. As your facial awareness improves, you will incorporate many newly learned practices into your daily habits. It will therefore not be necessary to repeat practising the movements you have already mastered because those improvements will have become part of a regular movement vocabulary. You will be doing them automatically.

Movement Vocabulary

Regular movement vocabulary is automatic. It's stored in the same way as in speech. When you are speaking, you don't need to look up all the words in the dictionary, or learn how to pronounce them: the word vocabulary is stored in your brain, ready to fit the context of your thoughts. Vocabulary is acquired by repetition. Hearing the same word and saying it over and over again imprints its meaning, usage and pronunciation into the brain.

Movement vocabulary works in just the same way. A repetition of controlled action trains small groups of muscles to work together and perform the necessary amounts of contraction or release to attain a desired shape. It's like moulding a new face without surgery, but with movement and breathing, feeling, deciding which action to take to achieve a desired effect — quite creative if you think about it, and the only tools you require are your eyes, brains, hands and a little sense of adventure.

I was once asked whether it was more difficult to learn a new move, or lose an old one; to condition or to decondition motor patterns. The answer is to educate the body like a child: if you take away something, give it an alternative instead. Then the loss is not mourned. So by adding new moves to your vocabulary and throwing away those you don't like, (instead of throwing away valuable skin as is done in a surgical facelift) you will improve the muscle and skin tone, you will look better, and with good looks comes confidence to get on with the things you want to do in life. A link will emerge between your inner feelings and what you actually expose to the outside world, or — even better — what you consciously choose to expose to the outside world. In this way your body and face can be used more effectively as a vehicle for living and communicating. You will be introduced to yourself as seen by an outsider.

It doesn't matter how old you are. It is never too late to become fully aware of oneself. Your self is your body controlled by your conscious mind. Your body is the most user-friendly machine ever invented but it is at the same time one hundred per cent alive. Like a machine it needs fuel (food) and maintenance (care and exercise); like any living organism it also needs oxygen, light and movement or change. Given these simple necessities, your body and your face won't ever look old and ugly.

Aesthetics and Feeling

The mere phrase "old and ugly" is exemplary of the basic misunderstanding underlying today's attitudes towards positive values such as beauty and happiness. Let me reverse these norms: consider a very young but extremely ugly screaming two-year-old with food and mucus smeared all over its face. The young are not always beautiful. Old and beautiful, on the other hand, is the memory of my 98-year-old grandmother waving goodbye for the last time at Budapest railway station. Against a background of silver-white hair, almost a century of summer sky blue poured out of her eyes, and tears poured out of mine as the train departed. Traditional concepts like "old and ugly" will soon fall apart when you have read this book.

Co-ordination and Toning

Co-ordination is the skill of moving. Movement allows blood and other necessary fluids to reach the smallest parts of the face and skin, thereby revitalizing their dormant state. The exercises in this book teach you that, given a little practice, almost any part of the face can move — yes, even your ears! Co-ordination and toning are intrinsically linked: if a body part can move, it is healthy and alive. If it is motionless, you are carrying dead meat around which hangs in an uncontrolled manner and forms a perfect bed for fat deposits and bags. So the more agile your face is, the younger and healthier it will look. Don't be afraid of moving the face because you think it might create lines or wrinkles. If the tone of the skin is healthy and supple, and the underlying muscle tissue fit to contract as well as relax, there will be no opportunity for wrinkles to develop. Wrinkles are river beds for tension. Eliminate the tension through movement and flow, and the wrinkle goes too.

Toning does not mean covering your face with the latest and most expensive cosmetic products. You will only need home-made natural ingredients, a little petroleum jelly, some herbs and oils and a few other fresh vegetables or dairy products found in any refrigerator. You will discover that your face can be mobile and expressive, that it can feel awake, fresh and happy on a purely physical level in the same way your body feels good after a workout. But there the similarity ends. The face and hands are often the only exposed, naked parts of the body. The face is the true self visible to others. Any movement, even the slightest, almost imperceptible, twitch reveals something of yourself to whomever you may be facing. It follows from further examining how the skin is linked to the underlying musculature that any improvement in small muscle control in the face enhances skin tone. An additional bonus is that the practice also embellishes expression and makes for easier communication.

Self-neglect and Surgical Facelift

If you are the kind of person who has an aversion to any form of exercise or physical practice, don't worry. You can do most of the exercises here sitting down comfortably in a chair or even lying in bed. They will give an unfit person a good sense of the connections between the brain and the body, and will trigger off a natural urge to move better generally. If you are the non-physical, let-yourself-go type, you are still able to survive because you can dress to camouflage yourself. But no make-up or surgical facelift will correct ageing disgracefully through self-neglect.

A surgical facelift is cruel, barbaric and doesn't make sense physiologically. What happens in a face lift? Untoned, flabby skin is stretched over fat and lame muscle tissue. The excess skin is then cut off, rejected, and thrown away. The skin on the facial area that has been "lifted" now has to manage distribution of vital fluids, air, water and blood through a reduced surface area. This is not going to help: on the contrary, most victims of this surgical malpractice have to go back after some time to lose more skin and the process continues until they have great difficulty in laughing, eating and even speaking. There is a limit to the skin's elasticity. The less skin you have, the harder it is to maintain it supple and healthy.

The Natural Face Book, on the other hand, values your skin. I wouldn't dream of throwing any part of it away. Each facial problem is dealt with systematically, one at a time. Yes, you will lose that double chin, but please keep your skin on!

Result

The result you want to achieve is a gradual integration of what you learn in this book into everyday life. You may well develop further exercises yourself to suit your own particular needs. The descriptions and goals to be attained are clearly explained and illustrated for each exercise. After the initial two-week introductory period, people will be asking you if you have been on holiday. As soon as you sink back into old habits, you will notice a slight deterioration in your face. But don't worry, progress always comes in waves. It may be hard but it won't be boring. As long as you come back to exercising, you will develop an awareness in your face throughout the day which will become natural and comfortable. You will know what your face looks like and portray your moods and expressions at will in a way that you yourself find pleasing and attractive. You will find that once you have started, there will be no return from a path towards a generally more pleasant lifestyle. The whole process is not easy, and you are going to have to work at it a little, but I promise you that you will enjoy every minute of exercising as much as I have enjoyed developing them. Soon enough, in a month or three, you will be using the exercises as an integral part of your daily routine for ever.

CHAPTER ONE

Self-Image

Confidence and Self-image

When I was running the dance studio, many women, much younger than me, whom I thought of as "young girls", would confide in me that they hated their bodies or were embarrassed about particular features. How depressing it must be to live inside a body that the wearer doesn't like. It soon became apparent at the studio that even the most unfit bodies could be made to look young and beautiful through the right kind of reconditioning movements. And as time went on, the regulars began to see rapid improvements and they began to like themselves better day by day. They changed from the whingeing weaklings who had first come into the studio, into confident, outgoing, pleasant people.

The first thing for you to do is to polish up your observation skills by watching others and noticing their posture and expression. Learn to watch: is the person upright, or are they stooped? Is their head centred on top of the spine, or are they carrying the head in front of themselves? Where is their gaze directed? Are they looking down at the ground? Where are their feet pointing?

When you see someone with an awkward posture, you will wonder if the person knows that they are walking like a hunchback. But of course they don't. The reason is that the person doesn't *see* him- or herself like that. Through observing others, you will become more aware of yourself.

In this way you will build up a more objective self-image. Do you remember how it felt when you heard your voice on a tape recorder for the first time? You thought: "I don't really sound like that, do I?", and it was hard to believe. Opening your perception to a more realistic self-image brings about a similar surprise. Physical development of any kind is at its most successful when you can regard yourself from the outside while feeling yourself from within.

Seeing yourself as others see you

How do you see yourself? Do you find yourself attractive? Are you popular and sociable? Are you introverted, shy or moody? What is your current self-image? It's not easy to draw up your own personality profile. Our self-image is the sum total of feedback we get from many different sources. The mirror is only one of them, and not a very accurate one at that. In fact, the image of the face you see in the mirror is a reversal of how you are normally seen by others. To get the picture that they see of you, place two mirrors at right angles to each other and look at the image in the second mirror.

Observation and Communication

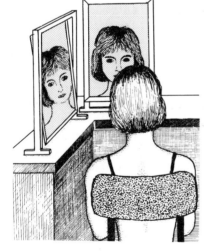

Fig 2: *Reversed mirror image*

Oh horror! On seeing a double reflection of your face you may suddenly notice for the first time that one eye is smaller than the other, one eyebrow lower, or one side of the lips sagging down. The other annoying thing you discover is that if, for example, you try to lift the dropped eyebrow, you find that you are moving the wrong one!

Two things emerge from this unpleasant experiment. Firstly, we seem to be used to or conditioned to the way we look. When we see ourselves every day in the mirror, the imbalances are just never noticed because they appear gradually, over a long period of time. Someone who hasn't seen you in 10 years notices the change immediately. There is some truth in the old wives' tale that if you frown when the wind changes, your face will stay like that for ever. Repeat an ugly movement enough times, and indeed, your face will acquire a piece of ugliness as a permanent feature.

Secondly, the failure to move the correct side when looking in an unusually placed mirror proves that motion patterns in the face are programmed partly through what we see in the mirror every day. This means that we rely on the familiar image of the face to locate its moving parts rather than sending instructions for movement directly from the brain into the parts we want to move. So the instruction to lift an eyebrow went to the wrong side when given to the reversed mirror image. The same awkwardness occurs when you try to move in front of a video camera, which also reflects the image twice.

Observation can sometimes be cruel but one usually learns something from nasty experiences. Imbalance in the face is the most ugly dilemma or facial problem, as you will see in Chapter 3. Don't worry — it can be corrected through the right kind of exercise. Having now already changed your self-image a little by looking into the second of two mirrors, what other surprises are there in store?

People around us, those we live and work with, give us a better clue about who we are than a mirror does. Their comments and reactions to our personality establish a particular self-image. As relationships change, so too does your self-image. Self-image is merely the facade of what you think you are, and what you think you are is what people around you make you feel about yourself. For example, I have a friend whom I have known since childhood. The change of personality of this single person throughout a lifetime is typical of many others. Such changes occur by chance or misfortune. My friend had a poor but happy childhood. She was outgoing and exuberant, always cheerful. As a young woman my friend was married to an alcoholic wife-batterer for six years. During that time she became withdrawn, introverted, shy and bad-tempered. Once that relationship ended and my friend was able to pursue her own talents and desires, she became her old happy self again. The moral of the story is: avoid bad company, and if you are confronted with it through circumstances outside your power, keep yourself at a distance. Never respond to aggression. Stay cool, and retain the image of yourself that you like.

But before you know which image of yourself you like, take a closer look at yourself. Take a look, for example, at your posture and your style of moving.

Posture

One can assess posture by the degree of comfort the body is in. If you are uncomfortable, then it must be bad for the posture. Sustaining an uncomfortable position for prolonged periods creates bad posture. Bad posture is not only ugly, it is also damaging to the body. Before you can have a positive self-image, it is necessary to see your negative one. Negative postural behaviour must be identified before any changes can take place.

Postural alignment

In order to see yourself in a subjective manner it is essential to know a little bit about posture, alignment, balance and direction. Our sense of beauty is linked by the laws of nature to physical competence, and comfort is synonymous with an aesthetically pleasing appearance: the two go hand in hand. Balance and comfort are determined by the ability to carry oneself against the pulling force of gravity. It is therefore not difficult to see how posture affects one's entire existence. To build up a positive self-image you may practise the following postural exercises. Begin by looking at your feet.

Feet

Feet placement

It is easy to forget that your feet carry your whole body weight when you are standing and walking. If your feet are not positioned properly, then nothing that is above the feet will sit correctly either, not even your head. Building a posture is like building a tower of child's building blocks. If the blocks are placed off-centre, they will fall down. The feet, being the base of the tower, must be the strongest and healthiest of all or they will suffer pain and be poor carriers of the rest of you. This is why placement and correct use of the feet should always be taught first in postural re-alignment. In fact, at the studio, every time a new client comes into class their feet are examined to make sure that the weight of the body is carried sufficiently well to perform the more demanding exercises.

Try to use the maximum amount of surface you have on the soles of your feet, including all the toes. Don't squash the feet into tight shoes, or you will be more likely to lose your balance. The bigger and broader your base, the stronger your stance will be. If your toes are squashed together and not allowed to spread out as they are designed to do to give maximum balance, then the weight of your body is being shifted backwards on to your heels alone. This means that when walking or standing you are very prone to being easily knocked over. The main two points about using the feet correctly in standing, walking and running are to a) spread the toes and b) divide the whole body weight equally between the forefoot and the heel. Compare the two footprints in Fig 3.

Notice how a foot enclosed in a tight, pointed shoe causes the toes to deviate from their natural position. When the big toe deviates from its alignment, its joint is traumatized by a pressing shoe, and a bunion develops. Squashing the toes together not only diminishes balance in the whole body, but it can cause bunions, hammer toes and all sorts of nasty foot conditions you can do well without.

If you are the type of person who thinks that high heels and narrow skirts make you look good, just bear in mind that you are projecting an image of vulnerability. This image has got women where they are today: the weak, vulnerable sex, still at the mercy of a more able-bodied man

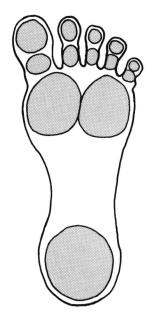

a) broad stance on bare feet
showing main weight bearing
points

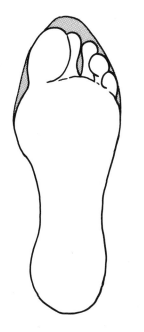

b) small stance on in tight shoes

Fig 3: *Footprints*

to help them out of taxis, wobbling on a pair of high heels, clutching on to a man and a handbag. In the aristocratic circles of ancient China, old women used to break little girls' toes, fold them under and bind them, to prepare them for a "privileged" life at the palace, as one of the Emperor's wives. Crippled for life, hardly walking and certainly not being able to run away from the Emperor, these young girls were assured, by this cruel custom, a future life of wealthy slavery.

There is no room here to write a whole book on what people have done to their bodies and their feet in the name of culture, fashion, image or prestige as opposed to health and comfort. It suffices here to say that for me, shoes are as much of a nuisance as bras, garters, hairpins, earrings, ties, hats, belts, bags, and a million other superfluous body items. Try not wearing shoes in the house and frequently play with your feet. Spread your toes so that they will all equally share the weight of your body together with the ball of the foot and the heel. Like the pads of a kitten, human feet are made for weight bearing.

If you follow the print a) in Fig 3, there won't be any danger of having common complaints such as flat feet. If your feet are already in poor condition, then now is the time to do something about it. And don't come to me with: "But my grandmother had feet like that — it's hereditary", because I don't buy hereditary factors. The philosophy behind this book, remember, is that you *can* change, whatever your age or condition might be, as long as you are willing to do something about it yourself, *now.*

From now on, you will no longer necessarily be sitting in an armchair reading this book. You will frequently be asked to stand up or lie down to try out a physical experiment or perform an exercise. So if you are comfortably lying in bed while reading this, close the book and go to sleep. You may start experimenting and exercising tomorrow, when you wake up. Set the alarm 10 minutes early to give you time. If you can't sleep right now, go to Chapter 7, page 111.

Experiment — Spreading your toes

Take your shoes off and stand on the floor with bare feet. Now try to spread your toes as far as possible. Make them look like ducks' feet. In the process of doing this, you will find that the fingers on your hands spread to accompany the effort made by the feet. This is because your brain is more familiar with sending messages to your hands than to your feet. Your toes are using a movement pattern that your brain already knows from when it sends messages to the fingers to spread. It is as if your fingers are trying to show your toes how to do the job, because the muscular contractions involved are of a similar nature.

The brain is such a clever organ that it will use whatever is already stored in its memory bank to cope with a new task. If, for example, you decided that you wanted to learn to write all over again, but this time with the left hand (that is, if you are right-handed), the task would be easier to you, already an accomplished writer, than to a child who is learning

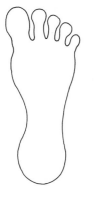

a) normal   b) flat feet   c) pigeon toes   d) high heels

Fig 4: *Human footprints*

for the first time and has never before known how to shape letters. The initial programming of movement patterns (as in the child learning to write) without pre-reference to existing similar patterns is hard, but once a pattern has been programmed into the brain, it will use every available previously stored pattern to aid in the development of new ones and thereby automatically rehearse its existing repertory.

When your toes are in their correct spread-out position and your body weight is carried evenly over your whole foot, without dropping the arch or deviating your big toe, you can learn to place the ankles and knees above the feet on your climb to rebuilding your posture.

Ⓑ Exercise No. 1   **Feet Placement**

Stand with the feet 12 inches (30 cm) apart, toes pointing inwards so that the big toes are almost touching, but the heels are kept apart as shown in (a) in Fig 5. Now keep the big toes in place and, over 10 counts, slowly close the heels without displacing the tip of your two big toes.

If your big toes are out of line, you will find this exercise almost impossible to do. In that case, reach down and hold the two toes together with a hand while bringing the heels together. You will have to sit on a chair if you can't reach your toes in a standing position. At the same time as realigning your big toe, keep the weight of your body on the front part of your feet, on the well-spread toes and especially on the big toes. This may pull and hurt a little but persevere through a small amount of pain. Now that your heels are together and your feet are pointing straight again, your toes should be more spread and they should bear more weight, so push the body weight forward over the toes, but without rising.

Stay there for a count of 20, breathing quietly. If it hurts a little, pull the toes out and apart with the hands and breathe deeply. One or two toes may give a little crack. That is very good for lengthening their joints and is totally harmless. When you finish, shake the feet out and repeat the

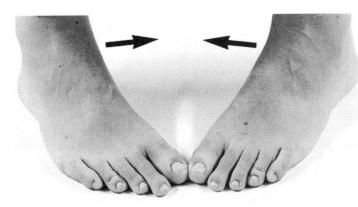

a) toes in   b) parallel

Fig 5: *Feet placement*

exercise slowly once or twice to see if you can make any other toes crack. Do this two or three times a week until you can crack all toes and stand with the big toes aligned as in (a) in Fig 6 without holding the toes with the hands.

Shoes

Before fitting a shoe, compare the sole of the left shoe with the sole of your right foot and judge for yourself if the surface area takes the shape of your whole foot. The shoe should have enough room for the toes to move and share the weight for your body in walking, jumping and running. Such a shoe is hard to find. Even the exorbitantly-priced jogging shoes usually lack a proper foot shape.

You should, within a fortnight, have changed the way you stand on your feet, provided you stop wearing harmful, narrow shoes. This will improve balance, confidence and strength in the rest of your body.

Ankles and Knees

Ankles and knees will be strong if a) your feet are broad and well-placed and b) they are properly aligned directly over your feet, with your body weight carried slightly forward, over the toes as well as the heels. Flat feet, whereby the body weight is carried on the fallen arch of the foot, makes for weak ankles that are sunken inwards, towards the mid-line of the body.

In their turn, they cause the knees to droop, and they are then in a weak position to carry the thigh bones, pelvis and upper part of the body weight, and so the gravitational chain goes on.

Ⓑ Exercise No.2

Pliés, Rises and Squats

Note: Plié is the most commonly used balletic term to describe knee bends. A demi plié is a bending of the knees while keeping the heels on the floor. A full or deep plié is the equivalent of a squat.

Stand with the feet slightly apart, feet pointing straight forward.

1. Demi plié. Bend your knees (keeping your heels on the floor).
2. Come back to standing with straight legs.
3. Now rise up on to your toes as high as you can.
4. Come back to standing.
5. Bend your knees again as in 1.
6. Do a deep squat (don't stick your bottom out).
7. Go back to demi plié as in 1.
8. Straighten your knees.

Fig 6: *Exercise No. 2*

Bend, stretch, rise, stand, bend, squat

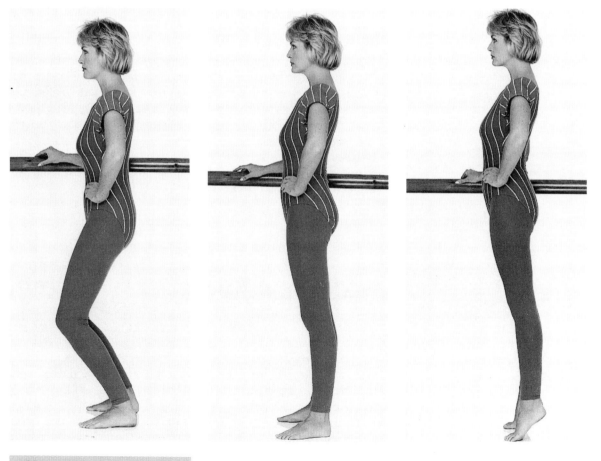

Practise the whole sequence once or twice a day. You can practise it when you are picking up something from the floor. This way of getting down is much better for the spine than diving to the floor with the head first.

A demi plié should get you straight down, without lifting your heels off the floor (this lengthens the Achilles tendon). When you can go no further, come back to standing by straightening your knees. On the rise, look down to see how many toes are supporting your body weight. Rearrange your toes manually, if necessary, if the little ones don't reach the floor. If you cannot do the full squat, hold on to a wall or the kitchen sink, and try to get down with your heels on the floor. Getting up again must be done with a straight spine and the shoulders relaxed, using mostly the thigh muscles and not the muscles of the spine.

The pliés, rises and squats give you all the vital leg movements for placing the ankles, knees and hips in a most efficient stance for strong support, good balance and grace. In addition, the squats are very good for your thighs and back muscles, averting all sorts of future troubles.

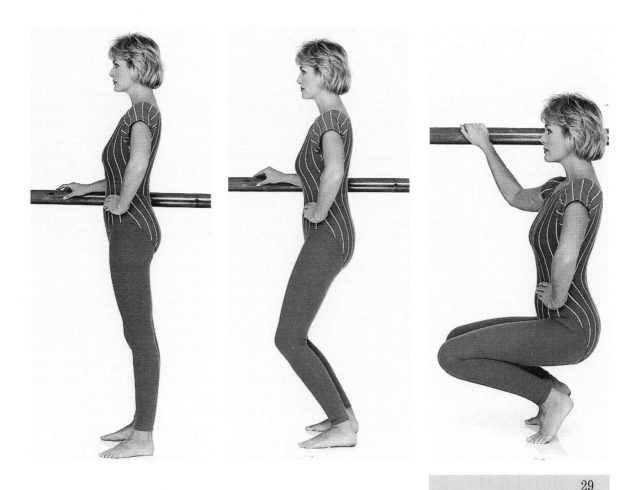

Pelvis

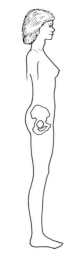

Fig 7: *The pelvis*

The pelvis is mechanically the most important part of the skeleton because it is in the pelvis that the centre of gravity lies, the point around which posture and movement are balanced. Correct positioning of the pelvis takes some understanding and practice and it is necessary for good posture to pay a little more attention to the pelvis which plays such a major role in the body.

The pelvis is like a forward-tilted basket sitting between the hips.

The basket contains your stomach, colon, liver, gall bladder, kidneys and everything else that is in there. It takes some effort against gravity, in the upright position, to retain the pelvis in a position which will keep all its contents inside. Some people have to make a conscious effort, at first, to keep the "tail" down to maintain a correct position. But as usual, effort is rewarded. If the pelvis is held correctly, you will suddenly discover that your fat belly has gone and, as an extra bonus, so has your protruding bottom. How come? Simple design mechanics. Compare the two pictures below and see for yourself.

Pelvic Placement

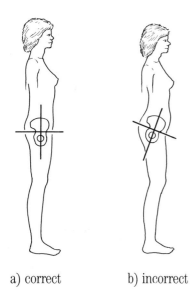

a) correct   b) incorrect

Fig 8: *Pelvis placement*

Stand up, facing sideways in exact profile to a full-length mirror, wearing nothing or something that allows you to see the shape of your body clearly. Your feet should be placed as in Exercise No.1: parallel, with your toes spread and the weight pushed slightly forward on to them. The knees should be relaxed but not bent. So far, so good. Your feet, ankles and knees could be seen as two strong, but flexible stands upon which you are now going to balance the rest of your body. The rest of your body is actually settled in the hip joints, supported by a large bone, the pelvis. At the back of the pelvis begins the spine. It is now absolutely crucial that the pelvis, which is, as it were, the second floor of the body "building", sits straight and does not hang to the side, forward or back, or else your spine, shoulders (which carry the weight of the arms), neck and head won't know where to go.

During the years of teaching average bodies at the dance studio I have noted, with interest, that while most women seem to suffer from the b) condition in pelvic imbalance, men, on the other hand, show the c) condition. Most men who came to class found it, at first, extremely difficult to sit on the floor with the legs and the pelvis held straight. They were sitting on the tail bone instead of the sitting bones (two protrusions at the base of the large pelvic bone, under your bum). The men didn't even know they had sitting bones. Apart from the short hamstrings, men's hips seemed stuck under the seat area, as if holding their bottoms very tight, contracting the lower part of the gluteus maximus (the buttock muscle).

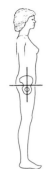

a) correct

b) forward tilt — belly down, bum up

c) backward tilt — pubis up, tail down

Fig 9: *Pelvic tilts and how they affect posture*

Here again, you begin to think: could that be so because men have had to wear trousers for so long, not being able to air freely what was most precious to them, their genitals? But you may come up with a better suggestion.

To assess the current position of your pelvis, look in the mirror and look at Fig 9. If your pelvis is vertical, as in (a), then you are fine. But if the pelvis is tilted as in (b) or (c), then you need to correct the alignment with one of the following exercises.

Ⓑ **Exercise No.3**

Pelvic Placement (1)

For a forward tilt (recommended for women).

To correct tilt (b) above, pretend you are a little boy who wants to pee further than his mates. Stand up, feet slightly apart, sideways to a full length mirror. Relax the knees.

1. Without sticking out your backside or tipping your spine backwards, thrust your pelvis forward 16 times.
2. Hold it in this position for 16 counts while squeezing your buttocks and tail tightly together.
3. Come back very slowly to the central position, as in (a), on 16 counts as well.

Don't tip your spine backwards. Look sideways into the mirror and check that the pelvis is tipped while the spine is vertical. The shape you are making should be like (c) on the illustration. Then come back to (a) while making a conscious effort not to stick out your bottom. Repeat once, but before doing so, turn around 180 degrees to check the alignment of your pelvis from the other side.

Ⓑ Exercise No.4 Pelvic Placement (2)

For a backward tilt (c) above (recommended for men).

Find a free wall somewhere and sit on the floor with your backside pushed right into the wall. You may bend the knees and push with the feet and hands towards the wall, until you can feel that you are sitting on your sitting bones. These bones can easily be felt by softly rocking from side to side in the sitting position.

1. Push forward from the base of the spine, working the backside back into the wall.
2. Push the belly button forward and down towards the floor.
3. Try straightening the knees a little.
4. Come back to sitting.

Check, by looking sideways into the mirror, that your pelvis and spine are straight in relation to each other. Feel as if someone is pulling the top of your head forward and upwards and at the same time come up to straight sitting again with a lifted spine and the shoulders relaxed.

Benefits of Good Pelvic Placement

Whichever way your pelvis is hanging, straightening it will help you in all sorts of ways. In women, having a properly aligned pelvis reduces the size of the belly and bottom. In both cases, a straight pelvis makes you taller, slimmer and stronger. Carrying the centre of gravity in its proper balanced position is, as explained earlier, much more energy-saving in daily movement, so you'll be able to do more and get less tired.

Waist Toners

The bone structure in the waist area is very thin. It is the place where the pelvis ends and the ribcage begins. The skeleton is wasp-like, only a few vertebrae thick at the waist. So women tended in the past to think that this area of their bodies could be squeezed for ever with girdles or belts, forgetting about the vital organs that happened to be inside. Today attitudes have changed somewhat but tight belts, elastic on underwear, and so on are still common practice and really hinder freedom of movement and respiration in the waist area.

It is important to keep your waist muscles supple and strong, as they are carrying the entire upper half of the body. Failing this, the body weight presses down on the thin bone structure of the spinal vertebrae. The following waist toners will soon correct the problem.

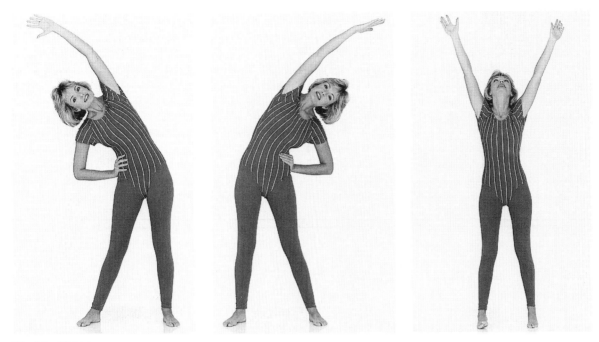

Fig 10: *Waist toners*

Ⓑ Exercise No.5

Waist Toners

Stand with your feet shoulder width apart with your hands on your waist. Make sure the shoulders are down and elbows out.

1. Make 16 side bends with one hand above the head.
2. Repeat to the other side 16 times.
3. Stretch upwards, rising up on the toes with hands above the head, looking up at the ceiling.
4. Slowly lower the heels and arms. Relax the shoulders and breathe.

Do this exercise whenever you feel lazy, heavy or tired. It will pick you up like a bouncing ball.

Ribcage

The function of the ribcage is to carry and protect the heart and lungs. The ribcage is expandable and with better breathing, it can become stronger. Whether you are happy about the size of your chest or not, whether you think you are too flat-chested or too well-endowed with bosoms, using the ribcage will work in both cases to your advantage. If you are skinny, the ribs will expand and if you are fat, good breathing and regular exercise will eliminate fat tissue.

How do you get rid of spare tyres? Fat tissue is always reduced when the underlying muscles become activated. It seems to be a rule that if a muscle is active, any fat tissue that may have covered it before exercise began just disappears. Fat is lazy, it doesn't like to move and feels uncomfortable lying on top of muscle tissue that keeps on moving about, so as soon as you start the waist toners, any spare fat simply vanishes. For example, if you find that your hips are too fat, just kick your leg 100 times a day into the direction of the lump of fat and the fat will simply go away within a fortnight. Since the friendly accommodating body's first instinct is to be comfortable, it is not going to keep a cumbersome lump of fat in a spot where that lump is in the way of movement. No, the fat won't go anywhere else either. It will just vanish into thin air: it will be absorbed and rejected by the body quite naturally.

For a slim, strong, mobile waist and a strong ribcage without any excess fat, do the following ribcage exercise.

(B) Exercise No. 6   Ribcage Articulation

Standing with your feet shoulder width apart with your hands on your hips, carry out the following.

Fig 11: *The ribcage*

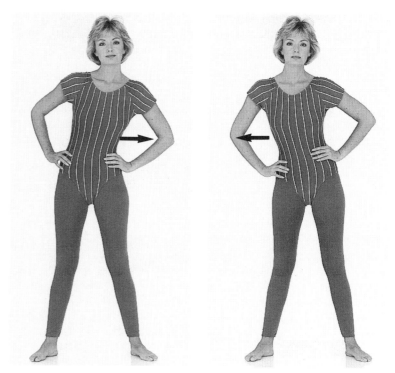

a) b) sideways isolations

34

c) d) twists

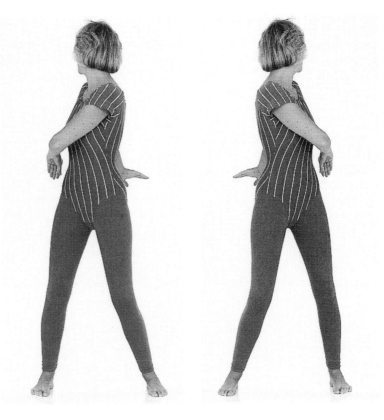

1. 16 side to side isolations.
2. 16 twists.

If you have trouble moving your ribcage sideways, stretch your arms out to the sides and pretend two friends are pulling your hands away from you, playing tug of war with your arms. For the twist, your arms should be loosely dangling by your sides and your head turned straight above your spine, your eyes looking back further than your body can go.

Make sure you keep the feet, ankles, knees and hips firmly facing the front, forming the strong scaffolding that supports your mobile waist and ribcage.

Benefits of a Mobile Waist and Strong Ribcage

When the ribcage is more free and mobile, breathing improves. Breathing is more important to the body than eating or sleeping. With better breathing patterns, fitness can only improve. Much backache and uncalled-for tiredness can be cured by waist toners and ribcage articulation as these complaints are, in part, caused by unfit waist and stomach muscles, leaving the job of holding the body in the upright position to overstrained back muscles.

Upper Back and Shoulders

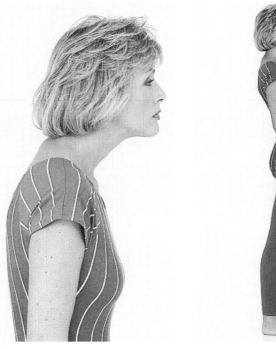

Fig 12: *Bad posture*   a) stoop   b) hollow back

When I meet people socially they often say: "Oh, you're a dancer, I'd better straighten up!" and their posture changes from a) to b) in Fig 12.

The most common error people make when they want to "straighten up" is to pull the shoulders backwards. The upper back and shoulders are the strong base for carrying your precious five kilo head containing all your thoughts and senses. The upper back must be kept broad and wide, with the ribcage expanded.

Ⓑ Exercise No.7

Loose Arm Swings and Circles

Stand with your feet in what dancers call fourth position: one foot in front, and one behind you while maintaining the pelvis (hips) in the central, facing forward position.

1. Swing your right arm eight times forward and back, making the movement larger and larger each time.
2. Carry on with the same momentum to make eight full circles, forward, or backward, whichever way your arm began travelling.

3. Speed up the circling motion until you can feel a slight tingling in your fingers. Spread your fingers.
4. Slow down, come back to half-circle swings. Hold the fingers high up above your head and shake your arm for a little while until you feel the blood circulating back down towards the shoulder.
5. Breathe, relax, change the position of your feet and repeat with your left arm.

Note: Please do observe the rest of your posture while doing these rigorous swings, or otherwise you are just getting puffed out for no reason at all!

Ⓑ **Exercise No.8** Shoulder Placement

Face sideways to the mirror, feet slightly apart. Now relax your arms and shoulders by the side of your body. If you notice that your arms are hanging slightly in front of your body, don't pull the shoulders back, as this will only narrow your upper back again. Instead, straighten your spine and leave your arms hanging loosely by your sides. Look into the mirror at the arm you can see.

1. Gently rotate the shoulder joint outwards, without lifting your shoulder, so that the palm of your hand comes to face outwards as illustrated in Fig 13.

Fig 13: *Shoulder placement*   a) dropped forward   b) rotating outward

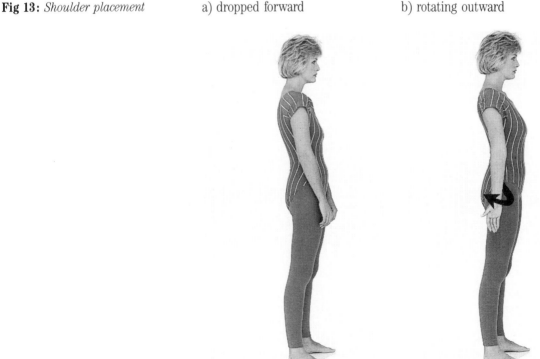

2. Let your forearms relax and mentally tell your shoulders that this is a better place for them.

Repeat the rotation eight times. Turn around and do it again with the other arm.

Once your shoulders hang freely in the right place they will no longer carry tension, and that is good news for the neck and the head. If your shoulders are very much out of place, do the above two exercises three times a week for a fortnight, then once a week for maintenance and your migraine and headaches will vanish for good. Further shoulder exercises are given in Chapter 11.

Head and Neck

The laws of gravity dictate correct positioning of the head above the trunk. In Fig 14 your neck is the pole, your head the ball.

It seems obvious that if this very heavy head (as heavy as five bags of sugar) is placed on a leaning pole, it is more likely to fall off. So if you don't want to 'lose your head' prematurely, you are well advised to rebalance it regularly with the following neck articulations.

Ⓑ Exercise No.9

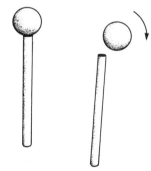

a) ball supported
b) ball falling off

Fig 14: *Carriage of the head*

Neck Articulations

The three basic moves for keeping your neck supple and strong are appropriately called "yes", "no" and "maybe".

Stand or sit with the spine erect.

1. Yes movement. Bend your head down and up 8 times.
2. No movement. Turn your head to the side 8 times.
3. Maybe movement. Tilt your head 8 times, keeping the tip of your nose in place.
4. Do a slow neck roll, rolling your head round both ways only once.

The above sequence should be done at least once daily, but slowly moving your neck, as many times as you need, will never do you any harm. More advanced neck exercises are given in Chapter 11, Shoulders, Neck and Chin.

The upper back, shoulder and neck muscles hold your head in its place. If you are able to balance your head on top of a vertical neck which rests on a well-placed spine as explained in the previous sections, then tension and effort involved in carrying your head will virtually be reduced to nothing. You will not only gain in appearance but also in saved energy. Hold the head back, on top of the spine, but don't lift the chin.

Posture in Walking

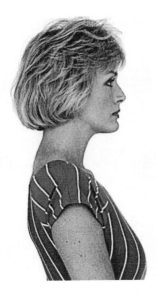

It is amusing to observe people walking and to notice a) where they carry the centre of gravity and b) which part of the body is leading them forward in walking. The following illustrations give some examples of the many variations encountered.

In walking, the feet are of course leading. Centrally above the stance is the pelvis, carrying the trunk which is correctly aligned above it. The neck should be held as an extension of the long spinal column, with the head balanced on top. Your gaze should be directed straight ahead or just slightly above eye level. Never look down to the pavement. This will make your head hang down and spoil your entire poise. Practise postural alignment every morning in front of a full-length mirror as you are getting dressed. Observe people's postures in the street. Are they carrying their heads on top of their spines? Where are they looking?

Fig 15: *Correct placement of the head*

a) forehead leads

b) chin leads

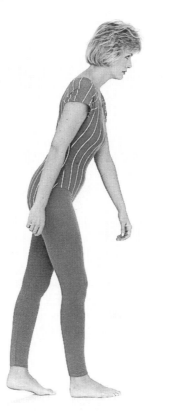

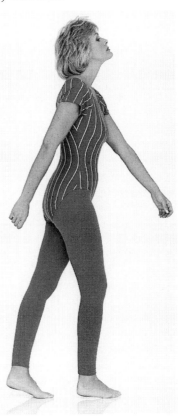

Fig 16: *Postures in walking*

Walking

Be aware of your posture as you walk. Keep your pelvis tucked under, lift your ribcage and hold your head high, but keep your chin down and look where you are going, not down to your feet or the pavement.

If it all seems rather self-conscious to you in the beginning, persist because the new feelings that you are adopting in your body will, sooner than you think, become just as natural as the old ones. They will not, however, be so uncomfortable for you in the long run. The key to a more positive self-image is comfort. The key to comfort is more efficient and balanced movement. It is important that the postural exercises are well mastered before embarking upon the facial exercises, as it is easier to change large movements and positions than small ones. All the exercises you have done so far serve as training ground for the latter exercises specifically designed for your face.

Fig 17: *Correct walking posture*

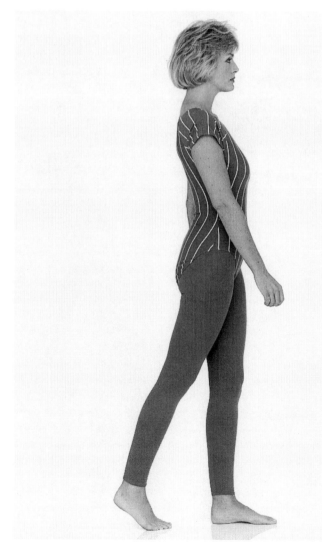

CHAPTER TWO

About the Face

The face can be seen as the mirror image of the soul. It works as a receptor for impulses and transmits messages. The face is the gateway to your personality. Know your face and get to know yourself better.

Where to begin? Start by watching other people's faces as they are talking, eating, sitting watching television or sleeping. Notice where they carry tension. You will find that while some people seem tense in the upper part of the face, around the eyes and the forehead, others will carry uncontrolled twitching movements in the jaw and chin area. Some people's faces are relaxed throughout; others display many unnecessary expressions, seeming almost hysterical. Watch the same person's face in different moods. When is it attractive, when is it ugly? The nuances between a smile and a cry, a whisper and a shout are so wide ranging. The trick is to find one's own boundaries and extend them each and every way. The exercises in this book teach you that static parts of the face and skull can actually move and be moved voluntarily by trained muscle action. The flesh on the face is akin to the soft clay of a sculptor. It can be placed and modelled with massage and exercise.

The Extended Face

It is hardly necessary to dissect the whole head to come to grips with the idea that the face is merely its front door mat. I am asking you here to

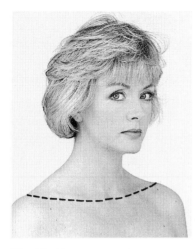

Fig 18: *The extended face*

deepen your vision and at the same time extend the size of your mat to a carpet, reaching from the crown at the top of your head to your clavicles (collarbone) and shoulder blades, not forgetting the entire back part of the skull and neck.

It is important to regard the face as part of the whole head. The hairline should not stop you moving and sending energy upwards towards the scalp. Regard the forehead, the scalp and neck as open channels for moving along blocked energy.

Like the body and the brain, the face needs change in life. The routines in this book are only some examples of how actions and exercises may be put together to form a balanced programme of facial activities. You will find, in good time, that your own feeling in the face will instinctively demand a certain treatment. Choose the exercises that you really like to do, the ones that really work for you. Take special care not to strain when you're exercising as this might have an adverse effect and extend your face in an undesirable way.

Relaxation

The skill of relaxation is unusual in that it does not involve using any special talent or effort whatsoever. Is your face relaxed now, while you are reading these pages? You will learn that good facial behaviour is a delicate balance between relaxation (release) and contraction to hold all the bits in the correct place. Your face is, of course, not fully relaxed while you are reading because if it was, then your jaw would be open and you would be dribbling all over the book — I hope that is not the case! To begin sensing various degrees of relaxation and contraction in the face, practise the following full facial relaxation exercise.

It's best to do the full facial relaxation at night before going to sleep but I often do one when I know that my face is very tense: for example, after an argument or if I am upset or angry. The full facial relaxation is always a wonderful remedy against irritation. Once you relax the face, problems somehow don't seem so bad.

Ⓑ **Exercise No.10**

Full Facial Relaxation

You will need:

- a flat surface to lie on
- two small cushions

Place the two cushions close to each other but not quite touching. Lie on your back, the nape of the neck on the spot between the two cushions.

Prop the little cushions (I sometimes use two rolled-up pairs of socks) tightly into the sides of your neck to stop your head moving from side to side. Pull the knees up slightly and relax your legs by dropping your knees together. The back of your neck and waist should be relaxed and not too arched. Rest the shoulders on the floor and keep the palms relaxed and open, facing upwards.

The secret about relaxing is to not feel any movement in the muscles, but to feel a very slow, passive, downward movement of gravity pulling on your body each time you breathe out.

1. Close your eyes, relax your eyelids and guide your attention towards the base of the neck. Take a deep breath in through your nose and breathe out slowly through your mouth.
2. Breathe regularly, and move your concentration upwards towards your jawbone and the inside of your mouth. If your cheeks are relaxed, your jawbone will drop slightly backward, down towards the floor.
3. Your tongue should be lying in the bottom of your mouth cavity. Concentrate in this area on the large muscles in the cheeks and again, let them relax on each out breath. Keep breathing at the same slow rate and now move your attention upwards.
4. Let go of all tension in your temples, eyes, eyebrows and forehead. If your closed eyes are restless and seem to be full of moving images, tell your eyes that it's dark now and that all they should see is black emptiness.
5. Feel your forehead expanding towards the floor as if the weight of your hair was causing the action.
6. Finally, relax your scalp and crown.

As you breathe out, imagine that your face is melting ice cream. On each out breath you will feel that the upper back and neck, the cheeks, ears and forehead come a little closer to the floor from sheer gravitational pull. Since you are lying supine, this particular pull goes in a favourable direction, towards the top and the back of your head. You can remain in this relaxed state for as long as 20 minutes or more. If you fall asleep, that's fine. Or you can come back to reality after a few minutes, but it is important to come out of relaxation slowly, not abruptly — use the regeneration exercise which follows.

Ⓑ Exercise No.11   Regeneration

You may do this exercise at any time when your body needs a boost. Lie down on the floor, close your eyes and relax for a few minutes.

1. Slowly open your eyes, taking a deep breath.
2. Stretch out your limbs, toes and fingers as if you had just woken up in the morning.
3. Slowly roll over on to your front and get up to standing, head last.
4. Now raise yourself on to the balls of your feet, and reach up with your hands, far up above your head, looking at the ceiling or the sky. Climb

with your fingertips higher and higher, looking up until you can grow no taller.

5. Finish by lowering the heels and, while sustaining a good stretch in the spine, lower your arms, and relax your shoulders.

When you are regenerated, you feel much lighter and more energetic.

The skin as a living organism

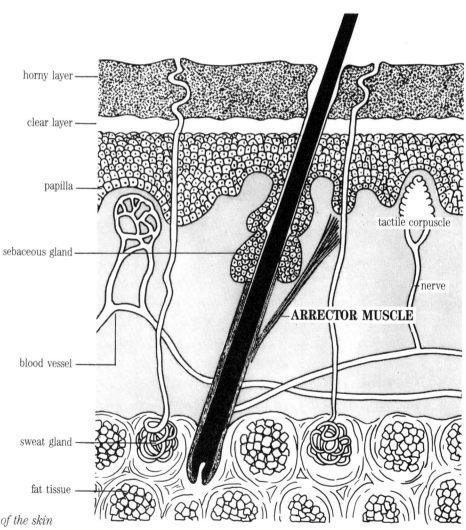

Fig 19: *Cross-section of the skin*

The skin has three functions apart from being a protective cover. Firstly, it is the organ of touch and feeling. Secondly, the skin works as a thermostat that keeps temperature inside the body steady. And thirdly, it rids itself of debris on a daily basis through sweating. Most of the senses we possess which make us aware of our environment lie in the fine nerve endings under the skin. The skin protects the body from outside harm, regulates the body temperature, excretes waste products, secretes juices (sebum) and sweat. The skin is the soil for hair growth and movement. A picture of a cross-section of skin looks almost like a seascape. The sea bed could be a muscle. Covering the muscle is a thin membrane of fat which could be seen as soft sand and soil. The skin could be seen from inside itself as a fibrous underwater jungle of hairs, minute muscle fibres, nerves, blood vessels, sweat glands, sebaceous glands, all growing abundantly towards the surface, the light. You can get an idea of the thickness of the skin by holding a hand with the fingers closed against bright sunshine and see the bright pink colour of your translucent skin.

Hair and Its Muscles

The hair root is implanted in a follicle (hair bed). Minute bundles of so-called involuntary muscle fibres called the *arrectors pilorum* cause movement in the follicle to alter the angle at which the hair stands on the skin. When you are cold the hairs stand erect to retain more body heat. To feel how these tiny muscle fibres work, do the following unusual experiment.

Experiment No. 2

Tiny Muscle Test

You will need:

- a small pan of boiling water
- access to a refrigerator.

Note: Don't do this experiment if you suffer from high blood pressure.

1. Put the pan of hot water on a surface next to the fridge.
2. Open the freezer compartment. Hold your face in or near the open freezer. Close your eyes and relax your face. Stay in the cold for 30 slow counts or more until your face feels really cold.
3. Still keeping your face relaxed, take the lid off the pan and quickly move your face over the steam. Don't go too close to the steam. Close your eyes and relax them. Breathe out through your nose.

A tingling sensation will rise all over your cheeks. This is caused by the movement of thousands of little muscles moving each hair follicle to adapt to the change in temperature. The power within these tiny little muscles is the secret behind the success of this face rejuvenation system.

Large muscles, such as for example the masseter (jaw muscle) are trained first to get rid of excess fat and to tone up the "sea bed". The skin is then fed with many delights and its little muscles trained to become voluntary, to do as they are told by the brain, in the same way the brains tells your legs to move in walking. It is a kind of miniature training programme to rehabilitate a prematurely senile, dormant face.

It is absolutely crucial that you relax the face during this experiment. It may be the case that, if you are unable to relax, you will not feel the action. in that case you should go back to "Full Face Relaxation" above.

Nerves

Are you too cold, too hot, itchy, in pain, or enjoying a caressing breeze on your face? As they come closer to the skin surface, the nerves grow and branch out. The nerve branches carry some *tactile corpuscles*, which means literally *touch bodies*, pushing up curiously towards the surface to tell you what to feel with the skin.

Blood vessels

The blood vessels dilate when you are hot, to let the warm blood rise up to the surface to cool off. In cold weather the blood vessels are contracted so that little body heat is lost. It is a good idea to rinse your face with cold water or iced water, to keep the skin tight and clean. Little red blood vessels, or broken capillaries emerging on the cheeks can be reduced to virtual invisibility by this method.

Sweat glands

Sweating has two functions: cleaning the body and regulating body heat. Impurities in the skin and tissues underneath are disposed of through sweating. Going back to the picture of the seascape, the sweat glands are at the bottom of the sea, buried under the sand. Out of each sweat gland grows a long duct up towards the surface of the skin. The sweat glands secrete water, salt and all the little bits of debris the skin wants to get rid of.

Sebaceous glands

The sebaceous glands owe their name to *sebum*, the substance they secrete. Sebum lubricates the skin to keep it soft and supple so that it doesn't crack. If the skin is exposed to a dirty environment, the oily sebum will pick up dust and dirt. In a clean environment it would be better not to wash the skin too much, as constantly removing the sebum with soap and water deprives the skin of its own natural lubrication. When the skin has to be washed a lot, "substitute sebum" is added in the form of creams, oils, lotions, and other moisturizing agents.

Skin care

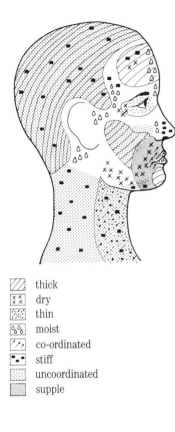

⧅	thick
x x	dry
⦂⦂	thin
◌◌	moist
⟋⟍	co-ordinated
▪·▪	stiff
⦂⦂	uncoordinated
▓	supple

Fig 20: *Skin types on one face: thin; thick; stiff; supple; moist; dry; co-ordinated; uncoordinated*

Dry skin

What to use to clean and nourish your face, and keep it supple, depends on a variety of factors. The cosmetics industry labels three skin types: normal, dry or oily. The truth is that skin changes type like a yoyo.

Firstly, your skin type depends on your ancestral roots — your genetic make up. Nordic people's fair hair and skin lets in more light than dark skin. Black or dark skin acts as a protective shade to keep harmful burning sun rays out. If you have a family history of eczema or poor skin condition, it is more likely that your skin will be sensitive too. Dietary conditions are most important as explained in Chapter 4, Clean and Feed. What you eat is what you are. If you fill your body with poisons, your skin will reject some of those poisons in the form of pimples, sores and other blemishes. Environmental factors also affect the skin. In a hot dry climate your skin can become very dry; in a moist, cold climate, stiff and tight. After a day in the city your face needs a sauna; after a day on the farm you are washing off "clean dirt". Your state of mind also affects the quality of your skin. Before I started exercising my face, whenever I got into an angry shouting match with someone, or had been very upset about something, I could count on the appearance of a cold sore on my mouth the next day as substantial proof of the poisonous words, thoughts and feelings I had experienced the previous day. Feelings cause chemical reactions in the body. In short, skin type is affected by genetic, dietary, climatic, environmental, and psychological factors. Different types of skin appear on different parts of the same face in varying circumstances.

Your skin is alive and forever changing. It is thicker on your jaws, forehead and chin than on your eyelids, lips and neck. The skin is thickest on the scalp. The nose and forehead are often sweaty and shiny in a warm room. Before a period the skin releases more impurities than usual, and a pimple suddenly appearing on the face is often a sign that you will be menstruating in a day or two.

Dryness is the biggest enemy of youth. When the skin is dry the face cannot move; it cannot laugh, eat or express itself clearly without increasing the depth of its lines. The movement limitations incurred through dry, stiff skin are the very cause of wrinkles. Poor nutrition, circulation and ventilation, and lack of light may all be causing unsightly blemishes on the skin. It is therefore obvious that putting on make-up is not, as a rule, something I would recommend. Yes, I can hear you saying, that's all very well, but what am I going to do about my red nose and those horrible little purple veins that cover my cheeks? Besides, make-up is pretty. Make-up is, like any form of adornment, fun and effective for special occasions but when adornment is applied routinely, it is no longer adornment: it no longer makes you feel special. You will find, as you proceed through this book, that your complexion and expression will improve amazingly. Make-up will become uncomfortable once the skin wakes up from its inactivity. Some make-up tips are given below. You will find some good face feeding recipes in Chapter 4, Clean and Feed. But before putting on your make-up, check for unsightly hairs on your face.

Unwanted hair

When I was performing in the dance company, I had to remove most of my naturally growing eyebrows to make space for stage make-up. Unfortunately, now that I no longer perform in the theatre and would love to have my original crop of thick, shapely eyebrows, they are, alas, still as thin as in my dancing days. Constant pulling out of the same hairs by the roots has stopped them growing back.

Really unwanted hairs, like those that stick out of the nostrils, on the moustache line or, worst of all, sitting on a wart or a mole, can be got rid off permanently quite easily provided they are pulled out slowly by the root. If the skin is moist and warm, extracting a hair like this won't hurt a bit. If you do it quickly and break the root the hair may be gone for a few days, but it will pop its head up again as in shaving. Treat each unwanted hair respectfully and keep gently pulling it out by its root. Eventually, after about 10 or 15 times, it will never return.

Make-up Tips

In Chapter 4, Clean and Feed, you will learn a completely new approach to keeping the face clean, supple and nourished. By treating your skin as a living organ rather than a painter's canvas, your complexion will improve to such a degree that you will no longer have any use for much make-up. You will use a mild soap only occasionally to wash off heavy dirt or make-up and the usual cosmetic products such as cleansing lotions, moisturisers, toning lotions, face scrubs and masks and so on will soon become redundant. In the meantime, use these tips when you wear make-up.

1. Massage cream or oil into the face about five minutes before putting on your make-up to allow it to draw into your skin. Gently wipe off any excess with a clean moist cotton flannel or natural sponge.

2. Only use foundation where needed. Look at your naked face and notice its natural colouring. Your nose and cheeks may be quite dark, while the forehead, jaws and chin are paler. Blend a very small amount of foundation only on those parts of your face that are embarrassingly purple-looking. If the colour of your foundation matches the colour of your "pale" skin on the other parts of your face, the result will be an even-coloured make-up base.

3. Never put foundation into wrinkles. Wrinkles in particular need moisture and air to be allowed to disappear. Chalky foundation or powder pushed into wrinkles is a bit like stuffing a pair of socks into a crying baby's mouth. It will not make your face look better; on the contrary, it accentuates wrinkles to fill them with cracking foundation.

4. No powdering. Powdering a sweaty nose will only block up the pores and make the skin more uncomfortable, less able to breathe. Think what it must be like to be a pore, sweating and gasping for air, and suddenly a huge dusty pillow is slapped into your mouth! No powder, whether it is loose or pressed, is going to help your skin in any way at all. To dry a shiny nose or forehead, just touch it lightly with the back of a clean hand which will gladly absorb some of that oily moisture: the back of the hands are usually too dry anyway.

5. Don't make ugly faces. Observe your facial expression while you are putting on your make-up. The following pictures illustrate this further. You may come across some familiar expressions: try to correct them.

6. Never go to sleep with your make-up on. Make-up is not recommended other than perhaps as a protective covering against worse damage from environmental devils such as stuffy nightclubs, town centres filled with car fumes, or dusty building sites. Of course, if you are going to a party, or performing an important public role, that's different. Just make sure it all comes off after the event. This book encourages your face to become so much healthier that soon it won't need a lot of make-up. The best way to get rid of make-up and prepare your face for the night is set out in Chapter 4, Clean and Feed.

Fig 21: *Putting on make-up*

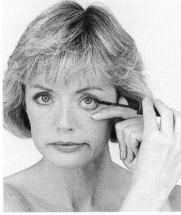

incorrect

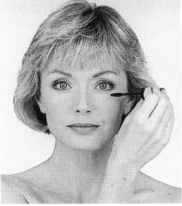

correct

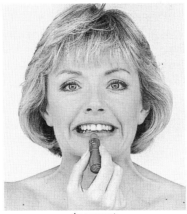

incorrect

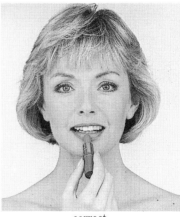

correct

49

7. Don't rest your face on the hands. When the muscles in your neck get so tired that you have to lean your head on your hands, it's time to go horizontal. Resting your head on your hands when sitting at a table, for example, will squash, fold and pull the skin of your face. Just don't do it. Lay your head down between two small pillows or on the floor instead.

Expression

While you are obediently practising the exercise routines, emotional feelings linked to specific facial expressions will emerge. You will learn to feel what it looks like when your face looks happy, angry, hungry, etc. Facial expression, the gateway to your inner feelings, will become known to your conscious self. For example, you could decide on a Monday morning to put on your "determined businesswoman's look" for an interview with a new client, while later that night, you may change your "facial dress" to that of a devoted lover for a rendezvous with your boyfriend. It takes more than clothes to make a woman (or a man). You will learn to economize on unnecessary facial movements while enhancing meaningful ones. Inevitably this practice will affect your mood and character. You will come to like your appearance better and as you do, your confidence will grow.

Managing expressions can make life a lot easier. It helps to be aware of what your face is saying, for so much mistrust and ill-will can arise from speech which contradicts facial expression. A friend may give you a compliment but have a frown on her face. The reason she is frowning may have nothing to do with what she is saying to you at that moment. She might have a headache, for example. When such facial expressions are repeated involuntarily they become ingrained, and an ingrained expression on your face gives false clues about the current state of affairs in your body. If you've just had a shouting match in a traffic jam on your way to the office and you don't manage to fix your face before getting there, your colleague will get a dirty look. What has he done to deserve that?

Unlearning Bad Habits

A good deal of this book is devoted to lifting these ingrained expressions, old maps which reveal every past tragedy. The facial exercise programme heals the scars. It feeds the superficial muscles with blood through massage and tones them through movement. The face unlearns these involuntary expressions by bringing feeling back into the slack or tensed areas. Hand-aided co-ordination exercises work tiny muscle groups into action without causing distortion. Avoid making ugly expressions and your ugliness will fall away. Imagine yourself shouting, spitting, coughing, trying to perform even the ugliest movements in a graceful manner. These movements will become so ridiculous that you won't want to use them very much. You will soon find out that a constant process of self-correction will help you work on your face. Learn one or two new exercises every day. Keep practising the ones you've learned until you can do them invisibly. In time, your face will always be worn with grace while you are getting on with the things you want to do in life.

In body exercise, when it is too hard or impossible to move a certain part of the body, like for example the ribcage, it is often recommended to use your hands as a guide until the feeling for the correct movement becomes conscious. Gradually one needs the hands less and less to achieve conscious co-ordination. In the beginning you will be so uncoordinated that you will be using your hands almost all the time to guide the muscles into performing movements that will, at first, be very unfamiliar. As you continue practising your face will eventually become supple, strong and co-ordinated enough to express a whole new vocabulary. To start with, though, you will find out that the sensitivity of your hands is crucial in this exercise programme. Apart from that, try from now on to observe the following list of do's and don'ts.

Do

- Eat a healthy diet made up of at least 75 per cent fresh vegetables, salad or fruit.
- Sleep in a dark, airy room.
- Keep your skin bare when you can and wash off make-up at night.
- Be aware of your expression at all possible times.

Don't

- Drink alcohol (as a rule).
- Drink strong black tea or coffee.
- Smoke.
- Indulge in nasty foods (red meat, artificially flavoured and coloured food, sweets, chocolate, cola, for example); if you've eaten or drunk too much, drink a pint of water to flush it out.

In the next chapter we will look at how to select your own individualized exercise programme and assess your progress. This list is fundamental to your face becoming fitter, fresher and younger.

CHAPTER THREE

Method, Assessment and Course Outline

Ugliness is merely a picture of unwellness. If someone is in a good mood and really healthy, then there is no reason why they should look ugly. An unfit, neglected face reflects trouble inside the mind and body.

Look upon regenerating your face in the same way as you would treat someone who is recovering from an illness. Spoil yourself with rest, good food, fresh air and exercise. Think positively and get rid of any fears or anxieties that you may have hidden in your subconscious mind. The body can best regenerate in a state of sleep or relaxation and massage. Illness and disease, infirmity, disorder, depression and the blues are all negative verbal statements describing a temporary problem: a pain, somewhere in the body. Locating and naming a pain or combination of pain symptoms creates a disease. This may help to cure it when similar pains recur, but classifying temporary pains makes them lose their passing state. They become recognizable symptoms which will be treated not for what they are, but for what their name stands for. So rather than treating, for example, drooping eyelids like a disease, an ulcer that needs to be cut out of the body by surgery, why not treat the feature as a positive challenge that can be overcome through the right kind of toning exercise? Exactly how this can be achieved is explained in the method of exercise that is unique to this system.

Method

This method is firstly to develop the muscles that can be moved and felt — the voluntary muscles. When these muscles are fully alert they can in their turn stimulate the surrounding dormant muscles which, in time, join in the action. Co-ordination power is thus multiplied with training. When all the dormant muscles have been woken up, and that takes quite some time, a whole network of tiny, small, medium and large muscle groups — sometimes reaching as far down as the shoulder blades and the centre back — all work together. You can then begin to feel the action of involuntary muscles. Once a muscle can be felt or seen moving, it can be localized by the mind, and the will to contract or release that muscle can be transmitted into it. In this way almost any muscle on the body can be made voluntary. The training programme in this book is based upon this natural chain of events.

Exercise Techniques

A single exercise usually causes one or more muscle units to contract, hold, and release. As the muscle contracts, it becomes hard and fills itself with blood. When the muscle lets go, or releases, it is soft, like a water-filled balloon.

Some of the exercise techniques involve very small degrees of muscle contraction. In order to use the whole range of muscle units lying on a particular section of the face, it is important to use degrees of contractions as well as full contractions. You could think of a muscle contracting step by step. Along the path of a full contraction from A to B are several steps or intervals. Each step has to be attained, felt and held briefly before you go on to the next step. This ensures that all muscle units are toned up individually as well as in harmony with each other. When the action has achieved its full contraction, when it can go absolutely no further and all the muscles involved are fully contracted and filled with blood, at this point of excruciating effort, they are told to remain in the contracted position for the same amount of time it took to get there and then to step down again, releasing the action little by little until full relaxation is attained. This must be accompanied by breathing and counting. You will have more fun practising to a favourite record and music will help you keep a regular rhythm.

Breathing and Counting

Breathing and counting are vital to exercise. I often practise to the radio in the car, or when I am working. Coherence of action, breathing and counting is shown in Fig 22. You will see that an exercise looks like a wave of energy, breath and rhythm.

Count	1 2 3 4 5 6 7 8	1 2 3 4 5 6 7 8	1 2 3 4 5 6 7 8	1 2 3 4 5 6 7 8
Breathe	in		out	
Action	contract	hold	release	rest

To feel the action of, say, your thigh muscles working in step fashion, in harmony with breathing and counting, try the following leg lift.

Experiment No.3

Leg Lift in Step Fashion

1. Stand by a wall or somewhere you can hold on to.
2. Now lift one leg just an inch above the floor, keeping the knee straight, and hold it for a count of three.
3. Lift it another two inches, and hold it.
4. Carry on lifting the leg like this, a bit at a time, for eight counts until it is at the highest it can go.
   Apart from the fact that this way of contracting the thigh muscle is most demanding, you can also feel that many different combinations of muscle work are involved in the process.
5. Hold your leg in its uppermost position for another eight counts.
6. Next — you are not off the hook yet — bring the leg down, step by step, in eight counts, just as you lifted it.

Effective Strength Building

When your leg is down again, the thigh muscle is most relieved. Relax and breathe to the rhythm of the exercise just performed and shake your leg about to release all tension. This experiment has shown you the tremendous power of the exercise technique which will later be applied to your face. This will, of course, not be quite as demanding as doing the leg lift in step fashion. In addition to muscle tone patterning, you will often be asked to assimilate a mental picture or visual image to help you to achieve the required results.

Visualization

Visualization helps to isolate small numbers of muscle units and make them work together. Auto-suggestive imagery (seeing things) and mind verbalization (talking to yourself) are not necessarily symptoms of insanity provided you do it consciously (at will) and for a purpose (training). So don't feel that it is silly to tell yourself that life is beautiful, or to imagine the smell of your favourite lavender oil, or that it is useless to pretend it's Indian summer in Massachusetts when you are sitting in Manchester on a bitterly cold and wet November night.

Use your imagination. Those grey clouds are covered with an immense blue sky and bright sunshine. Your eyes are not able to see it but your mind can and your mind controls your face, not the weather report.

Facial Muscles

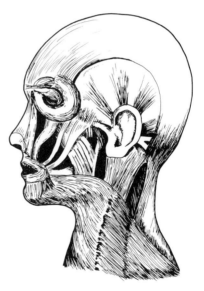

Fig 23: *The facial muscles*

The muscle map shows the main groups of muscles used in the face to help you understand how everything works. While practising, however, you won't be thinking in terms of muscles. Much more can be achieved by visualization of movement patterns rather than trying to figure out which specific muscle groups cause a specific action to occur. When a football player kicks the ball towards the goal, he has the goal in mind, not his thigh muscle. Especially in the relaxation exercises, visualization techniques are used to help you along.

Toning

Since, ultimately, the most visible effect of doing the facial exercises will be that the flesh on the face will be better toned, let us consider what toning really is about.

Toning the face is the ability to co-ordinate tiny amounts of muscle groups that will allow the face to become fit and expressive. To be able to tone up a certain part of the face, you have to be able to feel that part in isolation and then to move it in exclusion to any other part. Toning the face is a fine combination of gaining control over three different types of muscles:

1. Dormant muscles are muscles that are never or seldom used.
2. Voluntary muscles are muscles that we use consciously.
3. Involuntary muscles are muscles that seem to move all by themselves, without the owner noticing.

Dormant Muscles

A dormant muscle is a bundle of muscle fibre that is potentially capable of moving and therefore can tone up, but through lack of use becomes weak and uncoordinated to the point where it cannot be used at all. It becomes lame. Because dormant muscles never contract, never fully fill themselves with blood, they are very easy beds for fat to grow on. If a muscle is so weak that it is not strong and bouncy enough to protect the underlying bone structure from possible damage, then fat tissue comes along abundantly as substitute padding to protect the precious marrow-containing skeleton. Healthy muscles become hard (contract) when something threatens or presses against a bone. When the bone is safe, they relax. If muscles become weak and give insufficient protection to the skeleton then the body has to resort to the next best form of padding, which is fat. People who don't use their muscles often get fat. That is not a punishment, it is merely a safety device that the body is programmed to develop so that if you fell over, you would not so easily break your bones; fat tissue would catch the impact of the fall. A well-toned muscle serves as a soft bouncy cushion and no fat is needed on it. If the muscles on a person's backside are so weak that they cannot sufficiently cushion the seat area, then the area will grow lots and lots of fat to make sitting more comfortable for the body. If you don't want a big backside, just don't sit down too much. Toning the muscles in the face will eventually lead to toning the tiny involuntary muscles in the skin itself, making it once more supple, strong and healthy-looking.

The dormant face

Any flesh hanging loose on the face is dormant muscle tissue or fat. Muscle tissue can be toned up, back to its proper place. Once the muscle is firm, the redundant fat just disappears as it does on any other part of the body when it is exercised. Loose flesh folds easily, so when you are asleep at night the folds in your face are pressed into wrinkles. But don't despair — there are sleeping techniques explained later which will change all that.

If you are unfamiliar with any form of physical training, do the following exercise to make you feel and see the effect of voluntary movement versus involuntary movement. You will, while doing this, feel that your body can move at will if you make it move but that it will also seem to move all by itself, almost against your will.

Experiment No.4

Involuntary Movement: Wall Squeeze

You will need:

- a wall or door frame
- all your strength.

1. Stand sideways pressed to the wall or door frame with one foot against it, and an arm squeezed between your body and the wall.
2. Now with all your might, keeping the body straight and stiff, press your legs, body, your whole weight against the wall as hard as you can and stay there pressing harder and harder to a count of 60 or more.
3. When the pressure is most powerful and you really can press no more, suddenly step away from the wall leaving the squeezed arm hanging by your side lame and limp.
4. What's happening? Your arm is slowly and independently rising up in the air, all by itself. How does this happen?

It may seem like magic but in fact it's perfectly logical. The muscles in the recently-squeezed arm are still contracted from resisting the enormous pressure you imposed upon them. They were busy fighting the pressure to protect your arm from turning into an pancake against the wall, so your arm muscles were solidly contracted. When you suddenly removed the force, the power of muscle contraction in your arm lifted it up in the air. The muscles responsible for this action didn't get a message from your brain: they worked involuntarily. As you begin to become aware of unwanted muscle action, you can delete it from your movement vocabulary.

Voluntary Muscles

Voluntary muscles are muscles that are controlled by the owner's own conscious will. Typical voluntary muscles are the biceps, to lift the forearm, or the thigh muscle to make you walk. Most large muscles in the body that hold us in position and make us move are voluntary muscles. Don't forget that standing or sitting still also require a lot of muscular action, just to keep you in position. That is why it is not surprising when people who work at sitting jobs come home dead tired. It is more tiring to stand or sit all day than it is to have a mixed pattern of movement with some walking, lying, running, jumping and relaxing. Static effort or the holding of positions is the most tiring form of exercise, which is why it is used in aerobics, weight-lifting and other such torturing practices.

Most muscles started off by being involuntary or dormant. A voluntary muscle has learned to obey a specific command. For example, when you learn to drive a car, at first the muscles in the feet cannot co-ordinate the foot pedals but with repeated practice all actions can easily become voluntary, to the point when they become automatic. Before a baby can walk, his legs are involuntary (unwilling). But soon he is encouraged to put some will-power into the leg muscles, and, by trial and error, the baby will stand up, fall many times and try again until he is able to walk. **The transition from a dormant or involuntary muscle state to voluntary action is training.** The muscles of the tongue move when we speak and eat as they have been trained to do. Any muscle on the body can, with the power of will, be made to move. There is really no such thing as a voluntary muscle. A muscle has no will of its own. A muscle is just like a piece of raw steak. The power to move comes from the will, comes from you, the owner of the muscle, for only then has the muscle someone to listen to, someone to await instructions from. And since you are the boss in your own body, you should, with enough willpower, be able to move any muscle you jolly well desire. To feel how a voluntary muscle is made to move, try the following fist contraction experiment.

Experiment No. 5

Fist Contraction

You will need:

- a chair
- some attention.

1. Stand up and shake your right hand downwards until you feel your fingers getting hot with blood. Stretch your fingers and shake your hand again.
2. Sit on the chair and put your hand, palm up, on your lap and relax it.

Notice how nice and far the fingers open themselves naturally.

3. Make a strong fist and hold it, increasing the pressure for 30 counts or longer, until your nails begin to dig in to your palm.
4. Release the fist and notice that your hand stays half-closed for quite some time before it goes back to its original position. In fact, is it going back at all?

The speed at which your fist becomes a relaxed hand again depends on your physical condition: how tense and stiff or how relaxed and supple you are. The fist contraction illustrates how voluntary muscles work. They get a message to execute an action, contract and obey. But unless they get a conscious message to release, the lazy things seem to want to stay in a semi-contracted state for quite some time. This shows that even voluntary muscles behave in a way we are not always aware of.

Involuntary Muscles

Involuntary muscles are muscles that move without the owner's knowledge. Involuntary muscles can move perfectly well but they move seemingly all by themselves, without instructions from the conscious self. Involuntary muscle reacts to outside stimuli as, for example, when your hairs rise in the cold or when you suddenly scream if someone jumps on you from behind. This kind of involuntary muscle action is healthy and necessary for the body's own safety. But a lot of the time it plays tricks on you.

Involuntary Action

Because it is impossible at first to know one's own involuntary tics and twitches and poor postural or facial habits, it is better to learn to recognize them in other people. Observe people's behaviour in public places, on trains and at airports. You will see an entire spectacle of twitching feet, facial tics, ingrained expressions and nervous, fiddling hands. Involuntary action does not have to be movement — poor posture is part of it as well, such as an awkward gait, or bending down incorrectly to pick up a suitcase.

Self Assessment

Assessment of your facial qualities and faults will become an ongoing process of improving observation skills and intensity of feeling from now on. Look positively at your face. This will give you the courage to confront your negative points as challenges for you to tackle, rather than as life-long complexes which only weaken your self-confidence. The following charts are printed here for you to use as part of your training programme. Before scribbling all over them, take a photocopy of all charts. In a fortnight, take a fresh look at your face and compile your intermediate course programme. After that, I recommend that you use the charts at least once a month for booster courses until you no longer need them. So keep the originals in the book blank.

Positive Chart

Tick the features you possess.	✓
1 relaxed shoulders	
2 long neck	
3 evenly-balanced head	
4 full head of hair	
5 symmetrical hairline	
6 symmetrical (even) features	
7 good complexion	
8 smooth forehead	
9 clear, round eyebrows	
10 large, clear eyes	
11 long eyelashes	
12 good bone structure	
13 firm, happy cheeks	
14 a neat nose	
15 well-shaped ears	
16 well-shaped lips	
17 turned-up lip corners	
18 good teeth	
19 well-shaped jaw line	
20 other positive features	

Now that you have seen what the potential is in your face, look again and decide where you carry more tension: do you frown and tense the forehead and eyes? Or is the mouth tense and squeezed at the slightest disturbance? Do you belong to the "upper" or "lower" category of tension carriers? By marking the Exercise Charts on page 62 you will find out the answer to that question.

By marking the lines you carry, you can refer directly to the appropriate exercise in the book. Each exercise is marked by level: (B) for Beginners, (I) for Intermediate and (A) for Advanced. Begin with the beginners' level for the first two weeks of practice. Then take a week's break to get accustomed to new feelings in your face. By the beginning of the third week, you will be in a better position to reassess your face with the help of two mirrors. People will begin to compliment you on your looks in as little as two weeks after you start. Some of my clients felt that things got worse before they got better. That is a perfectly natural reaction to developing a more critical eye towards the face. When you begin exercising again on the third week, you may progress to the next level, but only if you are able to do the beginners' exercises that you selected well.

The exercises in the book follow an anatomical sequence. Having realigned your posture from your feet to your head in Chapter One, the facial exercises begin with the scalp and the top of the head, and work in the order of forehead, eyes, cheeks, mouth, jaw and neck, and so back to the shoulders. One of the best and most cruel ways to assess the current state of affairs in your face is to look at it upside down.

Ⓑ Exercise No.12   Upside Down Face

1. Stand in front of a full-length mirror with your back towards it, bend down from the waist completely and look at your hanging face through your spread legs. If you are past the age of 35, the initial image will be a shock to you. All the loose bits are now hanging the other way round. The top of your cheeks may almost cover your eyes. Your upper lip may lie dangerously near your nose. But you can also see that your double chin has gone and that you have a neck there somewhere.

2. All you have to do to get your face fit again is to learn to control all this loose flabby flesh and make the best possible use of it. This unattractive position makes you aware of the availability of the materials you have at hand to begin sculpting yourself a beautiful face. For the moment, gently shake your cheeks and try, in the upside down position, to contract your face slightly so that it takes on its more or less normal shape. The muscular effort in doing this locates all the areas you have to work on in the course of the exercises in this book.

3. Come back to standing and don't despair — when you look again after having exercised your face for a week or two it will already be much better, even in the upside down position.

To compile your own personal exercise plans, look up the exercise for each area to be worked on at various levels of achievement in the course summary charts which follow.

Exercise Charts

Level:	Beginners	Intermediate	Advanced
I. Upper Part — the forehead and eyes			
1. worry mark	10, 29, 30	13, 31	32
2. lines on forehead	10, 22-24	13, 31	35
3. frown	10, 30	31	34
4. crow's feet	10, 29, 30	31	39
5. small eyes	10, 36	37	40
6. puffed up eye lids	29, 37	36	16, 42
7. sinus blockage	10, 17	17, 55	16, 42, 56
8. lower lid bags	38	40, 46	42
II. Lower Part — the jaw and chin area			
1. flabby cheeks	48	45, 46	49, 55
2. hollow cheeks	46	50, 51	52
3. fat cheeks	45, 46	51, 53	54
4. moustache lines	10, 29, 30	56, 70	72, 73
5. wrinkled upper lip	66, 67	68	69
6. uneven lips	63, 64	51, 70	72
7. sunken mouth corners	66	65, 70	72, 55
8. annoyance mark	29, 49, 64	65, 70	71, 55
9. over bite	63, 64	70	71
10. under bite	63, 64	70	71
11. double chin	73, 75, 76	77	78, 79, 88
12. neck tension	9, 18, 22-26	27, 74, 81	15, 28, 78
13. short neck	9, 18	27, 74	15, 28, 78
14. lines in the neck	9, 18, 30, 73	31, 74, 75	15, 78
III. Other Problems			
1. headaches	1-11, 17, 18 22-26, 29, 36	13, 19, 27, 34	16, 20, 21
2. dribbling	53, 63, 64	65, 70	71
3. poor hearing	57	58, 59	60, 61
4. bad eyesight	36, 40, 41	43	42
5. lumps on the scalp	22-26, 29	19, 20	21
9. poor hair growth	22-26	19, 27	—
10. cellulite	14	—	—
11. tiredness	11, 29	13, 19	28, 61, 78
12. insomnia	10, 36, 44	81, 84	16
13. bad posture	1-9, 18, 44	74, 77	78, 82, 83
14. shoulder tension	7, 8, 85	81, 84	78, 82, 83
15. stoop	7, 8, 18, 73	74, 81, 84	78, 82

But don't be impatient — before you start leafing through the book for your favourite exercise, wait and find out in the following chapter how you can revitalize your whole head to prepare you for a radical change in your facial appearance. It is difficult to accept at first that you are going to be beautiful when you are not used to it, but don't worry, losing your ugliness literally feels like taking a weight off your shoulders. Preparing the whole head for facial treatment is more important than doing the exercises themselves, as all the energy you will require to understand and perform the exercises well comes from inside your head and will connect your face with your head.

Rules

1. Lubricate and Moisten the Skin

The skin is a very delicate organ. It is very important to lubricate your face with petroleum jelly or with one of the oil preparations suggested in Chapter 4. Otherwise, the effects of touching will be adverse and will stretch the skin instead of toning it. Always be very generous with cream or oil on your face. Never work on a dry face. Moisten the area as described above or, in an emergency, lick your (clean!) fingers before touching your skin. Your own saliva contains nourishing and germ-killing agents that are best suited to your body as they are "home produced". It's also free of charge and always readily available.

2. Don't Wrinkle

Don't wrinkle the skin while you work. The muscles of your face are going to learn to tone up and expand your facial movement vocabulary. They must not fold the skin that covers them. That is where your hands come in, to prevent the skin wrinkling during an exercise. Your hands will be needed until the point where very much smaller muscle units, so far unutilized, have learned to assist the usual muscles involved in an area.

3. Don't Stretch the Skin

Never stretch the skin. The exercises often refer to "pressing" gently. This is more like positioning the skin — it should never be pulled or stretched.

4. Don't Strain

If, at any time during exercising, you feel any strain or pain in the back of your neck, it means that you are not isolating the action but are using strength from elsewhere. As soon as you feel your neck straining, stop. When using your hands, push them against your face, not your face against your hands, as that is what causes the neck tension. A good remedy against this slight snag is to perform the exercises lying on the floor with the head supported until you no longer strain the neck.

5. Symmetry

Check with two mirrors on the evenness of both sides of your face as explained earlier in Chapter 1, Self-image. Always do an equal number of repetitions on both sides unless you can clearly see that one side needs much more practice than the other. In that case start with the poorer side, as one tends to put more effort into the first time an exercise is attempted.

Note: The hand holds illustrated here show only one way of doing an exercise. There are of course other ways and you may find that you can manage better with your own alternative hand hold. That is fine, provided you don't make yourself ugly elsewhere in your face while working on a particular area. It is very easy to pull another part of the face or to make ugly expressions while at work. Remember, the aim of these exercises is to lift your face up and make you more beautiful, not to turn you into a grimacing lunatic. Are you ready? Then let's begin!

CHAPTER FOUR

Clean and Feed

People spend so much time cleaning and grooming the outside of their bodies that they often forget what is going on inside. Unfortunately, many of us are often repulsed by the mere thought of anything to do with the inside of the body. But where else do most of the tarnishing impurities on your face come from, if not from within your own body?

Cleaning Inside the Body

When you have a close look at the body and how it all works inside, you begin to appreciate that all the intricate machinery we are made of must be vulnerable to abuse. Just consider how much work eating makes for your body, and while your stomach is trying to cope with unnecessary food, your energy level drops. If the stomach is never empty of food, excess leftovers will get stuck in the intestine and cause infections and internal swellings. Unfortunately, most social, romantic or business gatherings take place in a setting which involves excessive eating and drinking. In short, many of us force so much excess down our throats, it is inevitable that the body tries to reject some of it.

A lot of junk comes out through the skin. If you stick to a healthy diet without too much animal fat, or too many dairy products, and avoid all the other usual no-nos such as sugar, chocolate, alcohol, cigarettes, too much coffee and tea, there is no reason why your skin should be impure. I am not asking you to give up all your bad habits all at once, as long as you drink plenty of clean, fresh water after you have "sinned" to wash it all away thoroughly. As your body becomes cleaner inside, you will soon lose the urge to foul it up again. It's so easy: put less junk in and less junk will come out. Talking of junk . . .

Clean Up Your Act

Your daily waking up and cleansing routine involves actions of the most private and individual nature. What works for one person may not work for someone else. In this chapter there are a number of basic clean and feed routines to try out. In time, as you are able to do the other, more specific exercises, you will begin to incorporate them into these basic routines.

Here we are going to reverse the usual state of affairs — that you need to buy things to achieve goals. The first lesson in cleaning is to discard most of your collection of jars, bottles, tubes and other half-empty nasties gathering dust on your bathroom shelves and hidden in the depths of your bathroom or beauty cabinet. You may keep Nivea cream, petroleum jelly, some make-up but nothing else. For me, turning my back on cosmetic products began quite accidentally 25 years ago when I was a dancer with the Dutch National Ballet Company.

Heavy Make-up Removal

After every performance we had to clean our faces of heavy theatrical make-up, false eyelashes, wigs, glue, sweat and stage dust. Most of my colleagues had a large assortment of make-up removing creams, gels, lotions and moisturisers, with masses of cotton wool and tissues. I could never be bothered with all that and simply used to wash my face with running water and soap before running down to the canteen to catch my handsome boyfriend before he had time to impress any of the other dancers. My best friend and dressing-room mate was always telling me off: "Juliette, you shouldn't wash your face with soap — it's bad for the skin. You should use cleanser, toner and moisturiser. You are going to look old before your time." I felt very guilty, but at the age of 20, I found my boyfriend more important than sitting in front of a mirror for half an hour, rubbing bits of cotton wool and tissues in my face. A quarter of a century of more bottles and facial junk later, my friend's face is in no better shape than mine — in fact it's more the other way round.

For her, and so many others like her, who have spent so much money on cosmetics without real visible results, I have written this book. Today we know that rubbing your face with tissues leaves little bits of paper stuck in the pores of your skin. This stops it breathing, and like a fire, or a plant, skin dies without oxygen. Cotton wool is equally unpleasant on an everyday basis as it leaves tiny, invisible bits of fluff and minute hairs on the skin. Nowadays people are beginning to accept that it is O.K. to touch yourself, that it is not dirty or weird to use your hands and fingers on your skin. Care for your face with sensitive fingers, fresh water, some natural oils and nutritious products.

Ingredients for Cleaning and Lubricating

You will need the following:

- glycerine
- petroleum jelly
- fresh, clean water
- salt
- ice water
- two base oils (100ml bottles):

  1. Sweet Almond oil is for dry hair and skin on the face, rough hands and feet, and very good around the eyes at night against crow's feet and puffed-up eyelids.
  2. Wheatgerm base oil is rich in vitamins A, B & E and is excellent for neck wrinkles.

- Etheric or essential oils (30ml bottles)
- Three or four empty bottles to make your own preparations. Use not more than two drops of not more than five choices of essential oils. Add them to a 50ml bottle which is three-quarters filled with a base oil, to make a few different mixtures. Certain oils are good for particular problems, as shown here:

  Lavender: hair loss, insomnia, eczema, skin impurities
  Eucalyptus: mouth sores and weak gums
  Mint: headache, bad breath, toothache, colds, itching
  Chamomile: unclean skin, insomnia, mouth infections and a few

drops as hair conditioning rinse for fair hair

Lemon: greasy hair, rough hands and brittle nails, unclean skin, freckles

Orange: tired and flabby skin and wrinkles, pimples

Ylang ylang: sunburn, brittle nails, lifeless breakable hair, pimples

Sandalwood: blocked nose and sinuses, pimples

Geranium: non-serious burns and scars, throat and mouth infections, fever, eczema, unclean skin

Neroli: weakness, shock, nervous disorders

- Some plain soap
- White cotton flannels (don't use tissue or cotton wool)

Be careful where you buy the essential oils. They don't come cheap and must be got from a reputable source. Smell each oil and choose a few favourite smells from the above list. Don't worry too much about the healing properties given above; trust your own sense of smell. Train your nose to find the oils that are best suited for you, rather than looking at the information in too great detail. Choose the combination of oils that you most like the scent of; more likely than not, that will be the best choice for your face. Don't even buy the oils that you don't like the smell of. They are just not for you.

Remember, essential oils are very concentrated and quite costly preparations. Be careful not to put any essential oils near the eyes. Only use a few drops into the bottle of base oil/s and do not leave the top off for too long or your precious oil will lose its scent.

Massage Techniques

Two different massage techniques are used for different purposes: one for cleaning and one for feeding the face. The following diagram shows what routes to follow for a full facial massage, be it of the cleansing or feeding type.

Massage Technique No.1

Cleaning Massage

If you have been in a polluted atmosphere, such as in a traffic-filled city, or a smoky office, it is best to wash your face gently with a mild scentless soap first, just to get the worst off. After the initial wash you will need a preparation of one of the base oils scented with a few drops of essential/etheric oils (see page 67).

1. Before putting on any oil preparation you must warm up your skin with warm water or steam to allow the pores to open. Keeping the face

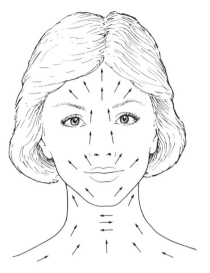

↑ Direction of movement

Fig 24: *The massage map*

warm, apply the oil mixture generously all over the neck and face, not forgetting the back of the neck, and if you can the shoulders too.

2. Starting at the base of the neck, between the clavicles, work your way up the face, moving the muscles under your fingers. The pressure against the skin must come from a right angle to the underlying tissue or bone structure so as to not stretch it (see Fig 25).

When you feel an unevenness on the face, a small piece of dirt or anything vaguely feeling like an unidentified foreign object on the surface of your skin, gently remove it. Your fingers' sensitive tips are better able to feel the surface of your skin than your eyes can see in the mirror. Trust touch as much as sight to discover the landscape of your face. The idea in this cleaning session is to remove dirt from the skin, so never press hard. Allow most of the work to be done by the body itself: your open pores excrete sweat and dirt. The movements of your hands should be like those of a mop on a wet floor rather than a scrubbing brush, or you might push dirt back into the vulnerably open pores. So instead of rubbing stuff into the face to clean it, you simply open the pores and let the skin excrete the dirt as it is programmed to do by the laws of nature.

3. When the skin feels warm, loose and slippery and you can no longer feel any impurities under your fingertips, take a clean white flannel that has been soaked in lukewarm water and wipe off all the dirt-containing moisture and oil. Use one surface of the flannel only once, then rinse off before touching the face again.

4. When the flannel no longer shows any signs of dirt coming off your face, splash the face with cold water and leave the skin to outdoor air. Even in the winter, your skin needs oxygen, so if it is cold outside, just open the window a little to let a cool breeze touch your skin. If you are worried about catching cold, wrap a towel around your neck and ears.

5. When your skin is almost dry, but not yet cold, put a little Nivea cream on your face, or one of the base oils (almond or wheatgerm) and gently tap the mixture into your skin with your fingertips until the skin is no longer shiny. Don't wipe the cream off with anything, but just keep tapping it in. If you have too much, use the excess cream on your hands, knees, the back of your elbows and your feet, until all of it has been absorbed by your skin, and none will have gone to waste on bits of tissue that are thrown away.

Fig 25: *Direction of pressure*

a) incorrect   b) correct

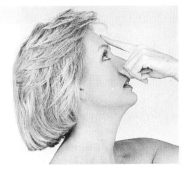
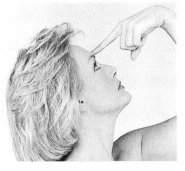

Massage Technique No.2

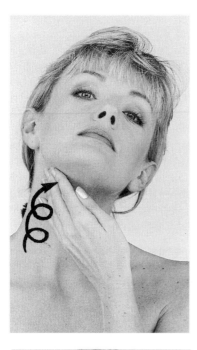

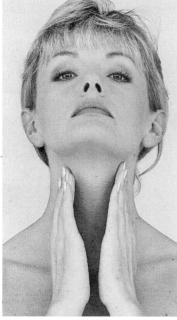

Fig 26: *Neck massage position*

Feeding Massage

About once a week, when your skin feels stiff and dry, treat your face to a feeding massage with one of the ingredients listed below.

For feeding:

- plain yoghurt
- cream cheese
- quark
- single or double cream
- cucumber
- carrot
- celery
- garlic
- banana
- avocado
- egg

Choose one of the nourishing ingredients just as you would choose a meal. Feel your skin and impulsively choose the first product that comes to mind. You may also use a fresh vegetable to massage your face. For example, a rounded-off piece of carrot gives an excellent eye socket massage, or even more refreshing is a fresh cucumber rub for your whole face.

1. Just lash it on. Press the substance, be it a squashed banana, a beaten raw egg or a handful of cream cheese, into the skin with your hands flat. Don't stroke your face or pull the skin with the food, just press it all firmly into the pores, not forgetting the temples, the area under the chin, the neck and the back of the neck.

2. When the whole face is covered, begin performing upward movements with your fingertips, again starting at the base of the neck. The position of the head illustrated below is recommended for neck massage. Stick your chin up and out, and make your lower jaw protrude until you feel that the skin under the chin is tighter.

3. Slowly work the food upwards into the neck. When you cross what look like rivers on the landscape of the face (wrinkles), give them the two wrinkle treatment exercises described below. You can also do these wrinkle treatments with your face oiled instead of covered with food. It makes no difference, and it is good to change. Following the routes on the massage map, continue working up the face, constantly moving the head and neck to provide contracted muscle tissue as a base for the massage. Continue like this all the way up to the hairline. In some places, particularly on the forehead and around the eyebrows, you may feel little sensitive bits which either protrude slightly or are slightly sunken. The hollow ones are acupressure points, the bumpy ones probably small pressure points containing accumulated sebum. Or you may come across a pulsating blood vessel, somewhere on the temple. Never press hard on a blood vessel or nerve: leave them well alone. In

time you will find it very easy to feel the difference between blood vessels, muscle, or fat tissue on your face.

4. Leave the food juices on for 5 or 10 minutes until your skin almost begins to feel stretchy. Then wash off with lukewarm water, no soap, and thoroughly rinse off with cold. You may like to tap your face with ice water at the end of a massage session to close off the pores and firm up the skin.

5. Keep the face supple after feeding. Before the skin feels dry again after a while, apply Nivea, or even better, sweet almond oil, this time on its own to keep your skin supple throughout the day. I have found that cosmetic moisturisers usually feel lovely when you first put them on, but their effect is not lasting enough. An hour or so later, the skin feels stiff and dry again. For ageing skin, the best moisturiser is a lavish handful of wheatgerm oil. If you think that it is too oily, try tapping the oil into the skin and dabbing with the back of the hand. It will soon be absorbed and no visible shine will remain on the face, only a feeling of supple mobility.

Ironing Out a Pressure Point

On some faces, there are little pressure points on the forehead and the scalp: little lumps of accumulated tension and sebum. These are often mistakenly referred to as acupressure points, which are hollow, more like little dimples. If you come across such a pressure point, treat it in exactly the same way as an acupressure point — with pressure. The only difference is that here, you should make a small circular movement while pressing.

① Exercise No.13   Ironing Out Pressure Points

1. Press the point fairly hard with your knuckles, or the back of a finger. Iron it out as you would get rid of a lump of flour in dough. Merge the hard little tension spot with its surrounding tissue.

2. Co-ordinate the pressure of your fingers or knuckles with a deep breath in through your nose as you begin to press. Hold your breath while increasing the pressure.

3. Slowly release the pressure and with it, let the air flow out of your mouth, ending the exhalation with a low sung note coming from the lowest part of your abdomen.

You will soon find that even after the first trial of this practise, the pressure points will get smaller and softer until, in a few days from now, they will disappear altogether, leaving your forehead free for more advanced reconditioning which you can find in Chapter 6, The Forehead.

Bath Recipes

When you are having a bath or a shower you can treat your face to unknown pleasures that may seem, at first, a little harsh or crude. But remember that if you want your face to be alive again, it is going to have to do some thorough training. So pluck up your courage and run a bath — not too hot — and add one of the following magic potions. Honey is very good for the skin and helps the oils to disperse in water. Cream or milk are also helpful against dry flaky skin. Treat yourself once in a while to a special bath by adding ingredients which will either help you relax at night or refresh you in the morning.

Evening Bath Preparations

To Relax Tension

1 dessertspoon full of runny honey and two or three drops of chamomile, sandalwood, orange and lavender essential oils.

To Stimulate Poor Blood Circulation

1 teaspoonful of sweet almond base oil, and a few drops each of mint, rosemary and lemon essential oils.

Cellulite

Cellulite is a ridiculous occurrence. Once again, I am afraid that the cosmetics industry has managed to advertise ways to get rid of a condition they invented themselves. Cellulite didn't exist until products to remove it were advertised, or at least it didn't have a name. I find it very difficult to believe that any cosmetic preparation would actually reduce cellulite. Cellulite is accumulated fat. Little babies have cellulite on their bottoms. Cellulite or fat is not evil: it is not to be feared. Like dimples in the chin or cheeks, fat can, with measure, in the right places, look rather appealing. You can't get rid of fat by applying cream to it. What you can do is to move more, sit less and stimulate and tone the body with massage and oils.

Ⓑ Exercise No.14

Abolish Cellulite

In the bath, you can apply rigorous massage to all the parts of your body that you find too fat. Feel and use the muscles under the fat and the fat will go away. So, if you are a victim of market creation, step out of the cellulite market into this exercise programme and never think about or even mention the word cellulite ever again. It does not exist. Accumulated fat tissue, however, does exist: if you have too much of it anywhere on your face or body, the following preparation has proved to be particularly good for massaging away accumulated fat tissue.

This bath is for when you wake up in the morning feeling particularly tired and lazy so you can't be bothered doing anything. Once you've done some stretching, breathing and toning exercises in this revitalizing bath, you will be as fresh as daisy again.

The amounts of oil given here are for a middle-aged skin in need of a lot of toning and feeding. Young bodies (under 30) can get away with teaspoonfuls rather than dessertspoons.

- 1 dessertspoonful of wheatgerm base oil and a few drops of lemon, ylang ylang, thyme and eucalyptus essential oils. Or try:
- 3 spoonfuls of single or double cream or some top of the milk and add two or three drops each of lemon, geranium, chamomile and neroli essential oils.

You may experiment further with making up nice bath concoctions as you become more familiar with the oils.

Bath Technique

There is hardly any point in having a bath unless you are going to go all the way and put your head under the water. If you are not used to this, now is the time to try it. Just lie on your back, hold your nostrils closed with one hand, hold your breath, tip your head under the water and relax. Your head feels light; it floats under the water, barely touching the bottom of the bath. If you need some air, just stick out your nose and breathe in; be a hippo.

Ⓐ **Exercise No.15**   ## Underwater Neck Roll

There is no better way of getting rid of a stiff neck than doing the underwater neck rolls, once you are accustomed to being under water.

1. Hold your nostrils (if necessary) with the left hand and slowly do a full head rotation towards the right.
2. Take a breath, change the grip on your nose to the other hand and repeat the neck roll slowly to the left.

   You may feel and hear some crunching in the back of your neck. Don't worry about that — it just means that things are moving again in that region.
3. Go down underwater again and now say "no", with your head, gently shaking it from side to side under the water. Try to stay relaxed while you shake your head loosely.

When you do this for the first time you may have just done one side and not feel like doing it again. That is fine, provided you start on the other side at the next opportunity. Training requires patience, no pressure.

Later on, you will be able to perform many facial exercises underwater and enjoy the benefits. When you get out of the bath, you will feel like you've just had a good dive in the azure waters of the Pacific Ocean. Your nasal cavity, sinus passages, ears, eyes and scalp will be clean, clear and express complete rejuvenation.

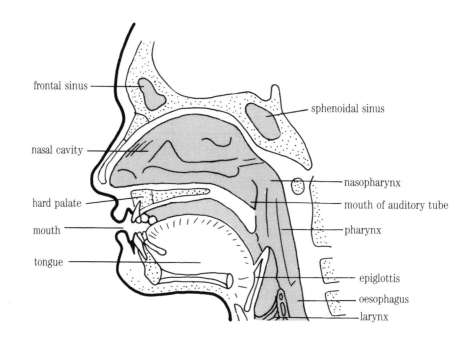

Fig 27: *Internal facial connections*

Nasal Cleansing

All the orifices in the body are connected with each other. In the face, there are channels going from the top of the nose to the eyes and back down the throat which also links the mouth to the ears.

In order to keep your major faculties (sight, thought, smell, hearing, and voice) working for you in the most efficient way, it is important that their connections are kept clean and free of blockages because they rely on each other for individual functioning. To feel the connection between the ears and eyes, for example, stand on one leg and close your eyes. You will fall over. The apparatus for balance works on principles of gravity and movement of liquid in the inner ear. Of course, sight also helps to locate your whereabouts in relation to the space around you, and the two together keep you in balance. If you eliminate one, by closing your eyes, a strong readjustment of awareness is required before you can balance again as effectively as with both faculties in function. In this way your senses work together to keep you happy and healthy.

This is why the nasal passage cleaning exercise, although quite unpleasant at first, is important. I assure you that you will even enjoy it once you have become accustomed to it and experienced its refreshing cleansing value.

(A) Exercise No.16

Cleaning the Nasal Passage

1. Bend over a sink filled with salted lukewarm water and take some water in your cupped hands.
2. With one nostril at a time (that means closing off the other nostril), breathe in a little water. Take care not to swallow it or let it enter your windpipe!

You have to deal with what happens next in your own way. The aim is to get rid of sinus blockage, mucus trapped in the nasal cavity and other dirt sitting in the very top part of your nose. Your job is to get it all out of there.

Keep alternating between the left and right nostril until you are able to pass clean water all the way from the nostrils to the throat. Be careful not to swallow any dirt or that will make you sick. Spit out the dirt, cough it out, sneeze.

(B) Exercise No.17

Ear Popping

1. Press your nostrils and eyes tightly together, close your mouth and blow.
2. Press inside your head outwards. You will feel your ears popping.

Don't worry, your head won't burst. When you have finished with this rather violent practice, hold your head in its balanced position on top of the spine and gently shake it from side to side again as if you were saying "no", and breathe a little deeper than before.

Other Underwater Exercises

At a more advanced stage, almost all the exercises given in this book can be performed underwater provided there is no soap or other eye irritant in the bath and the breathing is mastered. A little milk or honey can even be soothing.

Massaging the scalp is another of my favourite bath exercises but it is better if you learn to perform a scalp massage outside the bath first, before washing your hair, with a home-made mixture of sweet-smelling and nourishing oils as described in the following chapter.

CHAPTER FIVE

Healthy Hair and Scalp

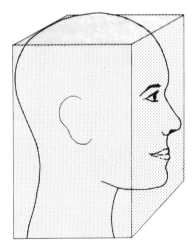

Fig 28: *The head as a cube*

I have already explained that the face should not be treated in isolation, like a mask. If you can imagine the whole head as a cube, then you will see that the face merely occupies one out of its six surfaces. The temples, under the chin, the back and top of the head form the remaining five.

Many massage and exercise techniques given in the following chapters involve movement energy that flows up into the temples, hair, scalp and skull, far beyond the actual boundaries of the facial "mask" itself. If, like other books on the subject, we had treated the face as merely one of the six surfaces on the head, the results of this exercise programme would not have been so complete and long-lasting. Because the face is part of the head, as the head is part of the whole body, it is not possible to begin working on the face itself until you have felt and exercised the whole head, including the skull, scalp and hair, as a living and reacting part of the entire self. You will need a full awareness of the position, functions and connections of the face in relation to the whole head and the rest of the body, in order to achieve the astonishing results that are possible with the methods in this book. If talking about cubes and geometrical surfaces sounds too scientific and academic, why not turn it into a living landscape?

Facial Landscape

Imagine your face to be a flexible landscape which covers the entire skull, the back of the neck, and upper back and shoulders. On the front side it

76

starts at the clavicles (collarbones), the upper ribs and the breastbone. Like a stocking pulled over the skull, the whole area is one. The hair growing on the scalp could be imagined as a healthy forest on a mountain top. The mountain top, hard and rocky, carries the soil for the growth of your hair, the scalp. Beneath the rock is your brain. Your eyes could be two lakes, your cheeks the undulating hills halfway down the valley. Your nose, ears and mouth could be deep caves, leading to the innermost depths of your geographical being, hiding like geysers and volcanoes the powers within you. So you see, the face doesn't just stop at the hairline, the chin or the back of the jaw. In fact, movements in the face often project themselves throughout the body, and vice versa.

Our facial expressions and everyday facial movements (eating, speaking and so on) are affected by muscles as far away as the lower back and the abdomen, even the legs. Ordinary tasks we perform in our everyday lives affect the movements on our faces.

There are several factors that make your face twitch or move involuntarily. Notice how your face will cringe with involuntary movements in a crowded room full of such background noises as kettles boiling, children screaming, or dogs barking. Concentrating hard can have the same effect. Try, for example, putting down a mug full of tea down on a hard table without making a noise. The sheer concentration of executing a difficult movement often causes facial muscles to contract in an odd way. A young child is beginning to formulate the shapes of letters on paper when learning to write might stick her tongue out with concentration. As an experiment in sensing connections between different parts of the body personally, do the following exercise.

Balancing the Skull

The postural alignment of your body varies from standing up to lying flat on your back.

In the standing position the spine is slightly more curved, to carry the body weight which is pressing down and supported entirely by the soles of the feet. In lying, where the body weight is distributed evenly throughout the skeleton, the curves are not really needed at all. No bed has yet been made with a dimple for the skull instead of a pillow, but logic has it that the skull should be, as it is in children, centred above the spine so that when a person is standing upright and holding the head in the correct place, they should not be able to see their feet, or any part of the body for that matter. Several images may be given to help you improve positioning of the head. The first one, which I was given as a seven-year-old at ballet lessons, was to imagine a piece of silver thread attached to my breastbone lifting me upward towards the sky. The object was to induce a classical ballet posture of lifted ribs with the neck held tall and high. Although the image may be useful for growing children, it would be inappropriate to use it as an adult. The image I prefer to relate to is the one where the weight of the body is pulled upwards from the crown. Oddly enough, if you hang a person upside down by the ankles on a machine called the a gravity invertor, the natural drop of the bodyweight indicates that the crown coincides with the line of gravity.

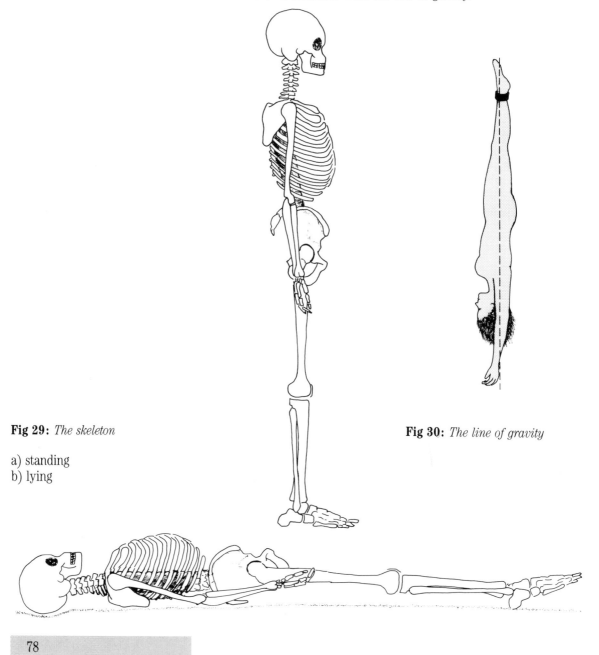

Fig 29: *The skeleton*

a) standing
b) lying

Fig 30: *The line of gravity*

Ⓑ Exercise No.18

Head Placement

1. Stand with your feet slightly apart, with your knees relaxed and your pelvis straight.
2. Lift your ribcage and relax your shoulders.
3. Place your neck centrally on this structure by pulling the back of the neck backwards and keeping your chin down.
4. Your head, which is resting on the atlas (the first vertebra in the spinal column, situated between the earlobes) is now able to balance with minimum effort. It was a revelation to me that the centre of gravity for the head was so deep and so high. You should be feeling as if your crown were pulling you up; your gaze should be slightly above the horizontal. In this correct position, your eyes should not be able to see any part of your body. If you can see your knees, thighs or bust, it means you are leaning forward.

Note: Some of the exercises given below to liven up your scalp, and thereby improve the quality of your hair and tone of the neck, chin and shoulder region, may seem slightly rough to you. However, training requires strength, daring and risk-taking. Don't shy away from touching yourself for fear of hurting yourself. To touch is to heal, and as long as you perform the exercises intelligently, according to the instructions, there is no need to worry.

The Scalp

Working on the scalp is, like working on the forehead, extremely revitalizing. If your scalp is neglected it could become the home of much headache and migraine misery.

Scalp massage is a good way to get rid of tension which might otherwise lead to headaches. To make a scalp massage really enjoyable, choose one of the preparations listed below, depending on the present condition of your hair. Make up only a small cupful of a preparation which you will only be using once. Make enough to wet all your hair. Mix them and heat up to a temperature as hot as your scalp can bear, and carefully pour over your head. Massage your scalp vigorously and cover up with a polythene bag or cling film; leave the mixture on for at least 10 minutes before thoroughly washing out with a mild scentless shampoo.

Nourishing Scalp Massage Oil Preparations

For Dry, Damaged Hair

¼ cup olive oil and
¼ cup of cod liver oil

For Fair Hair

¼ cup of sweet almond base oil
add a few drops of
chamomile, lemon and rosemary essential oils

For Dark Hair

¼ cup of wheatgerm base oil
and a few drops of
lavender, sandalwood and ylang ylang essential oils

For Dandruff

¼ cup of sweet almond base oil
¼ cup of strong sage and thyme tea
1 dessertspoon of runny honey
and a few drops of eucalyptus and rosemary essential oils

Massage Technique No.3

Scalp Massage

1. Sitting on your sitting bones (see page 30), with the spine erect, begin behind your ears, at the base of your neck.
2. Put your two thumbs there, with the other fingers resting on your temples.
3. Now slowly push your fingers through the hair on your scalp. Of course, the main sensation is that you encounter hair, but forget about that for a moment. Concentrate on feeling your fingertips gliding along your scalp.
4. Gently move your hands up until all your hair is gathered on a spot where you might have had a ponytail as a child.

Now feel if there are any lumps, crusts, soft bits, hard bits, warm bits or itchy bits. How varied is the floor of your scalp? When you come across an area that needs scratching, resist the urge to scratch for a moment. Instead, firmly press your fingertips into the area and take a full deep in breath while doing so. This action will free the flow of energy in that area, as opposed to merely scratching its surface. Move your fingers in a circular motion. Be careful not to trace your fingers along the skin but to keep them in one place and make the underlying skin and muscle tissue move over the bone. At the back of the neck, at the base of the skull you might find some lumpy bits of permanently contracted muscle tissue. The idea is to go to the base of such a tension spot and push it out of the way (just as you would knead a lump of dry flour in the dough when making pastry) until it blends in with its surroundings and disappears. Slow, deep breathing should always accompany the ironing out of tension spots.

The direction in which the lumps are massaged away has little relevance, as the idea is simply to merge the tension spots with the surrounding matter and allow them to spread so that fluids and blood may once again flow through the area freely.

If you have no bumps and lumps at all, then concentrate on those areas that are the most sensitive to touch. If an area feels as if it doesn't want to be touched at all, that is the place needing most attention. The common headache as we know it in the West is largely caused by these tension spots which have accumulated from stress.

Stress and Tension

Sometimes clients at the studio suffer from emotional problems which appear to be caused by emotional stress. It usually turns out that physical treatment eliminates the problem instantly. What happens is that people are in pain but because they cannot identify or name the pain, they create verbal, emotional problems to explain their unidentifiable discomfort. People tend to relate the word stress to mental, psychological or emotional problems, when stress is in fact a result of purely physical muscular tension and rarely anything else. All over the Western world, we are advised to learn to relax, but the very nature of our competitive and money-orientated system is inconsistent with relaxation. Stress costs Western nations a fortune in health care. Yoga, relaxation courses, masseurs, therapists, osteopaths, and meditation retreats are all trying to help people overcome the daily stresses of modern life. I personally believe that this Catch-22 situation could be resolved by simply changing immediate environmental needs; beginning with the removal of a million unnecessary objects such as most pieces of clothing, accessories and furniture which all hinder freedom of movement, and make us subconsciously feel "trapped".

Tension or stress can arise from physical discomfort. If the body is not comfortable it will use muscle groups to aid in supporting its uncomfortable position. I could always tell from looking at a person's posture and gait, as they walked through the yard into the studio for the first time, what their complaints were going to be. The migraine sufferers usually carried their head in front of them and a shoulder bag hanging from a permanently raised shoulder. One woman always held her right hand closed while doing exercises. I asked her why, and she said "That's where I always hold my car keys."

If you tend to suffer from headaches, it is probably due to accumulated tension. Next time you have a headache don't swallow any tablets. Instead, lie down on the floor and do some of the exercises described in this chapter. Tablets merely hide the pain from you, making you unable to get rid of the headache naturally. Migraine sufferers who swallow painkillers regularly have reached such a permanent state of tension and hidden pain that the condition has become chronic and, if treatment with pills (numbing agents) is continued, will only get worse. A further disadvantage of painkillers is that most of the tablets disturb the digestive system with their distasteful sugar-coated acid and bitter contents. So in addition to headaches, you may develop stomach ulcers as well. Throw away all your painkillers and begin to feel your pain. There is nothing wrong with pain. Pain is a warning that something in your body needs special attention, that's all. Listen to your body and converse with it through feeling, massage and movement. In this way you will soon be able to deal with any form of pain in a rational, intelligent way, without immediately running to the medicine cabinet or the doctor. Of course, if the pain persists and you don't understand why, then you should go and see a doctor.

Tension in the scalp may come from a number of sources: hairpins, elastic bands, hats, glasses, harsh lighting, noise, or polluted air. It may also come from the way you hold your head and from a lack of free movement in your neck and shoulders. Having tension or being free from it will depend on the degree of control you are able to exert upon muscular habits throughout the whole body. When you have finished exploring the landscape of your scalp, try some of the following exercises, all of which will revitalize your scalp and encourage healthy hair growth.

Ⓘ Exercise No.19   Scalp Knock

This exercise is particularly helpful when you are tired but want to carry on working for a while. It will really give you that extra boost of energy and take away a lot of tension in your head. You can do the scalp knock at any time, in any position.

1. With your knuckles, gently tap all over your scalp and compare all the different sounds you can produce with your voice while doing so. The speed and vigour with which you want to do this is left entirely up to your own feeling. You will find that some places on your scalp feel painful at first.
2. Continue tapping for a while, move to a different area, then come back to the sensitive spots. The pain will gradually disperse.
3. Continue knocking the knuckles of both hands on all the hard parts of your skull until you feel like stopping.

Ⓑ Exercise No.20   Horizontal Head Butt

You will need:

● a carpeted floor space
● a folded-up towel or flat cushion.

The head butt may be performed lying down flat on your back, on a carpeted floor, with your knees slightly pulled up, in the usual supine position. Your hands should be resting under your head. Support your head with your hands as if your head was a foreign object, a dead weight.

1. Lift your head just ever so slightly with your hands; quickly remove your hands before the neck muscles get a chance to contract and let your head drop on the floor.
2. You may repeat the action only as many times as you comfortably enjoy after having tried to do it right. Finish the horizontal head butt by gently rolling your head from side to side on the floor, breathing slowly and relaxing.

Note: Don't lift your head up too high, or you might end up with a concussion!

The benefit of the horizontal head butt is that if it is performed with good timing the impact releases spasmed muscles in the neck so deep that they cannot be reached with massage. Revitalizing your scalp is the most effective way to release migraine tension.

Ⓐ Exercise No.21   Upright Head Butt

This exercise is for more advanced students. You can do it on your own against a wooden or cork wall. You can do it with a partner, using their head instead of a wall which makes for a fun game (but caution is advised, as bumps incurred are your own responsibility).

1. Starting with the hardest part of your skull, the top part, gently knock your head against a solid surface. Expose different areas of the skull to the sensation of a gentle head butt and notice the differences in intensity of feeling, hardness of the scalp surface etc. in different areas of your skull.
2. Don't repeat so often that it hurts. The sensation should be surprisingly pleasurable with a soft bang but no pain.

When your scalp has regained its vitality through massage and movement, we can begin considering the hair.

Types of Hair

The cosmetics industry wants us to believe that all the millions and millions of people's hair neatly fit into one of three categories: normal, dry or greasy. The truth is that on one individual's head, there may be as many as seven different types of hair growing.

Starting at the back of the neck, at the base of the skull you will find firstly some very thin hairs. Further up, the hairs become thicker. Pulling on these hairs is very sensitive, as they are connected to tiny nerve cells.

Moving upwards towards the ears, the hairs become more sticky, warm and greasy from sweating. Going up further towards the top of the skull we find that the hair becomes more sensitive again when it is pulled. At the very top of the skull where we find areas of hair that are thick and abundantly growing. This is the area that most benefits the "head butt" described above.

Healthy Hair

Healthy hair has weight. It moves like the sails of a ship or the soft grass in a wind-blown field. All the exercises here will improve the quality of your hair and will benefit the muscle tone and skin texture of the scalp. In addition, they will tone up the neck, and help to reduce any double or triple chins that you may have. Always brush with the opposite hand from the side you are working on. This allows the muscles on the same side as the brushed area to relax fully while you are brushing. Treat your hair to a good brushing several times a day.

Ⓑ Exercise No.22   Sideways Brushing

Hold the brush in your right hand and bend your head to the right side.

1. Brush your hair from the left of the base of the neck, from behind your left ear and temple towards the crown. Drop your left arm as if it were dead and relax all the muscles in your left shoulder and the left side of your neck. Feel the stretch in your neck and, gently lifting your scalp upwards with each brush stroke, guide the movements towards the top of the crown.
2. Do 20 brush strokes then rest.
3. Repeat on the other side, this time tilting the head to the left and brushing with the left hand. If this proves awkward, do 30 strokes instead of 20, to get used to it. You will soon learn to use both hands evenly.

If you have problems switching hands, go back to the co-ordinated hand, observe how the brush is held and how the movements are performed, then switch on to the clumsy hand and copy the actions exactly in mirror image.

Give the right shoulder and arm (or the left if you are left-handed) a good rest while training the clumsy side to become active. Ambidexterity — the ability to use both hands equally well — is a key to rebalancing the body, and we are never too old to learn.

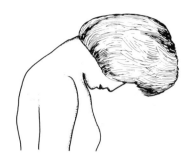 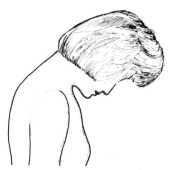

Fig 31: *Back of the neck tension*   a) chin rests on breastbone   b) chin does not reach breastbone

Ⓑ Exercise No.23

Forward Brushing

Bend your neck down as far as it will drop, with your chin touching the breastbone. If your chin does not reach your breastbone (with the jaws closed, otherwise you are cheating) it means that you are carrying tension in the back of your neck. In fact, the amount of tension carried in the back of the neck and shoulders can be measured exactly by the distance between the chin and the breastbone when the head is dropped in this forward, relaxed position. The degree of neck tension can be measured by the inch.

Don't worry for the moment how far your chin reaches down. Frequent repetition of this exercise will soon loosen the muscles in the back of your neck to allow the head to relax fully and drop downwards. When your head is truly relaxed in this forward hanging position, you should feel the skin and muscles in the back of the neck, and the muscles in the upper back pulling. They will, with more practice, become longer and allow the head to drop down fully until your chin is resting on your breastbone. Keep your shoulders relaxed. Your free arm should be dangling down, completely relaxed.

1. Using one hand only, begin to brush from the base of the back of the neck, working upwards towards the crown, the top of the head and towards the forehead.
2. Do 25 strokes with one arm, rest, breathe deeply, then repeat on the other side with the other arm.

Ⓑ Exercise No.24

Backward Brushing

Stand up, lift the chin and look up towards the ceiling or the sky without bending your neck too much.

If your neck muscles are not strong enough to hold your head back without resting it in "the lap of the shoulders" (a no-no in good postural behaviour) then you may support the head with one hand while brushing with the other.

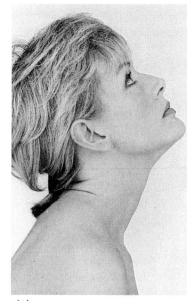

a) incorrect

Fig 32: *Bending the head back*

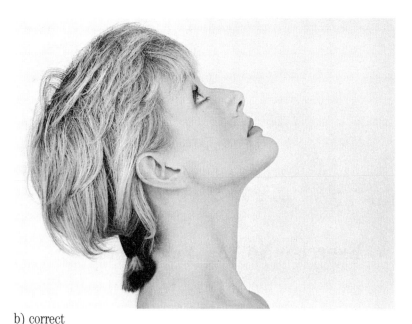

b) correct

1. Brush from the hairline upwards, towards the crown.
2. Stick your tongue out as far as it will go.
3. Now say "oooo" and smile at the same time
4. Make 20 strokes with one hand, change hands and repeat on the other side.

Keep your chin lifted, open your eyes wide, look up high.

Sticking your tongue out tones the underside of your chin, as the base of the tongue is attached at the angle between the chin and the neck.

The above three hair brushing sequences are a clear example of how an ordinary daily action can be transformed into a healthy routine which deals with several problems all at once, without necessarily spending any more time doing it than you would normally. The brush strokes benefit the neck line, double chin, scalp, temples, back of ears, and eyes. When you are familiar with all the other exercises that follow, you will exercise automatically during every morning freshening-up routine. You will no longer have to think about it.

The Crown

The brush strokes also benefit the crown. All directions for hair brushing as described in the previous three exercises lead towards the crown. With the help of two mirrors we shall try to locate the exact location of your crown. Some people claim to have two crowns. For a fit face, one crown is quite enough, provided it is in the right place. Ideally, it should be situated where the centre line of gravity passes through the uppermost point of the skull. Imagine the top of your head as an open umbrella. The crown is its peak, and the handle should be your neck and spine. If you find that your crown is not centred, or too low, this may be caused by incorrect carriage of the head and neck and will be remedied as soon as you improve your posture.

Even if your crown is not in its place, put your index finger on the uppermost part of your skull to feel where your crown should be situated. Once that spot is known to you, you will be able to guide your daily actions in brushing your hair and massaging the scalp towards this point and, believe it or not, within a few weeks, your crown will have moved to its correct position, placed centrally at the uppermost tip of your skull. The body, in its usual friendly manner will be only too willing to place your crown where it is meant to be.

It is interesting to note that both in acupuncture and in yoga the crown is a vital point of energy source, so obviously it should be well centrally placed. In yoga the crown is the top chakra, guiding vital external energies, coming from high above the physical body, directly into the system. Carrying the crown in its correct place is a vital part of feeling centred and lifted.

Ⓑ Exercise No.25   Hair Shakes

To cover the maximum range of movement possible in the neck, shake the head in three separate moves, eight times each. The moves are again called "yes", "no" and "maybe", to cover the three planes of movement.

Fig 33: *Hair Shake*

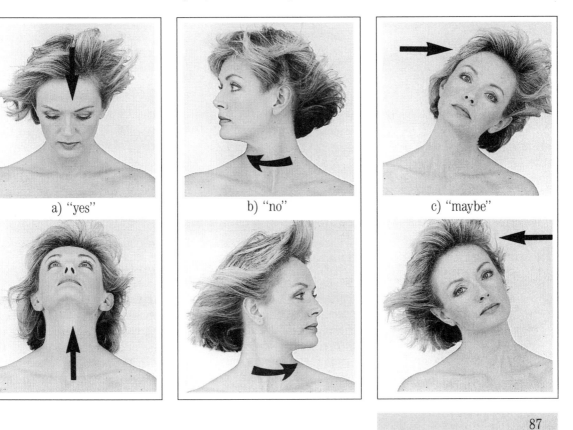

a) "yes"   b) "no"   c) "maybe"

Ⓑ Exercise No.26   Circular Hair Shake

1. Slowly look around the periphery of your vision to achieve complete head rolls but bear in mind the position of the neck as you bend back. Again, if your head seems too heavy to hold around the back, use the hands in support.
2. Repeat twice to each side.

Ⓘ Exercise No.27   Upside Down Hair Shake

An easier way to do circular neck movements is to let the whole body hang down from your waist so that your head is somewhere between your legs. You may bend your knees a little if your hamstrings are too short.

1. Relax your neck and the shoulder of the arm you are not using.
2. Rotate your head loosely and shake your hair down and out while brushing at the same time.

Ⓐ Exercise No.28   Figures of Eight

The figure of eight, which I learned from my children, is a fantastic rebalancing exercise, not only for the head but for the whole body.
Stand firmly with the feet slightly apart, and drop the head down.

1. Keeping the face down and relaxed, begin slowly making a continuous loop of figure of eight shapes in the horizontal plane. As you reach the lowest part of the movement, you feel the full weight of the head pulling down. With each lift towards the sides, the weight diminishes to release the muscles on the opposite side of the neck. Get into a regular increasing tempo until the movement is mostly made by momentum, rather than muscle force.
2. Continue making the shape and gradually increase the speed of the motion but don't go too fast. Carry on until you reach a pleasant sense of rhythm, harmonized with the speed of your breath. Do not do more than about 15 repetitions in the beginning or you might feel a little dizzy.
3. Take a rest and breathe, and find your bearings before repeating the exercise an equal number of times the other way round. When you have done a good number of fairly vigorous figure of eight loops and still manage to stand up firmly without getting dizzy, it means that you are well balanced.

The benefits of all head shakes, but especially the upside down ones, are improved blood circulation, thereby increasing blood and oxygen supply to the brain, and improved balance. It will also move the hair wildly in all directions and thereby stimulate its roots and follicles to create a stronger and healthier scalp.

Note: If you have trouble with low or high blood pressure, these exercises will be very useful. But start them slowly and gradually. As long as you always make sure you are standing firmly on bare feet and **come up**

slowly from a downward bend, these should not make you dizzy. There is nothing really wrong with getting dizzy, but dizziness can make some people afraid, and we are working for strength and courage here. In slow motion, the figure of eight may also be used in the treatment of poor hearing both as prevention and cure (see Chapter 9, The Nose and Ears).

Hair Growth

The way in which hair is implanted in the skin looks like a plant rooted in the earth. The quality of your hair reflects the state of health of your body. Hair growth varies from one part of your head to another. The hair on the top of your head grows faster than the hair behind your ears. It is possible to locate areas of poor hair growth and stimulate them with massage to increase blood flow as a preventive measure against balding.

Hair is attractive and feels nice when it is long enough to flow and move in the wind. The underlying skin, the "soil" for hair, should be humid and well ventilated. Like a plant, hair cannot live without water, light and air. There is no reason why hair should not grow abundantly at the rate of between one and three centimetres per month. Any amount of excessive hair loss is due to one or a combination of three things: 1) state of health in the rest of the body, 2) how the hair is treated, and 3) hereditary factors. Good health includes a balanced diet. Poor diet, excess smoking, alcohol and caffeine will seriously damage the health of your hair.

The second cause is, as usual, abuse. Hairdressers, like doctors, have to make a living. If people treated their own hair, hairdressers would be out of a job. What happens to your hair during a perm or a colouring session is not very pleasant. A perm burns the hair. Colouring uses heavy chemicals like peroxide, ammonia and many other poisons to get rid of your own natural pigmentation, and then adds artificial colour to replace the lost pigment. The colour of natural hair is not even. Dyeing the hair makes it look artificial and bland. It is really best for the hair if it is allowed to keep its natural colour and texture. Grey hair may be rinsed with henna for brunettes and with strong chamomile tea for blondes. This makes the hair healthier, is harmless and will make you look young again.

Whatever the state your hair is in right now, begin to give it some personal attention. You may go to a good hairdresser just to have that super cut once in a while, a cut that is shaped to enhance your facial contours and allows your hair its weight and movement, but avoid at all cost having it artificially coloured, permed or straightened. Feed your hair and massage your scalp instead. You will soon find that your hair is not that bad after all.

Hair Washing — How Often?

Hair should be washed as often as it needs. As your scalp, hands and general ability to feel your body improve, you will find out when your hair needs washing. It does not make sense to say once a week, or once a day. Hair quality is affected by environmental conditions, in the same way as the rest of the face and the body also has its own cycles. About a week before a period, for example, the body is very busy rejecting debris and your hair can often be greasier at that time. The following infusions may be used as hair rinses to stimulate hair growth and improve shine. Use them cold, after washing your hair, leaving them on for 5 to 10 minutes with some cling film over the head to prevent evaporation. The recipes given here and above for scalp massage (see pages 79-80) are only suggestions. You may like to experiment for yourself with your collection of oils and tea to develop a preparation that suits your own body.

Hair Rinse Preparations

For Fair Hair

¼ cup chamomile tea
a few drops lemon and eucalyptus essential oils

For Dark Hair

¼ cup henna
a few drops geranium and rosemary essential oils

For Dandruff

¼ cup sage tea
½ teaspoon sweet almond base oil
a few drops rosemary and lavender essential oils

For Balding Hair

½ teaspoon honey
½ teaspoon wheat germ base oil
a few drops orange, eucalyptus and ylang ylang essential oils

For Greasy Hair

for blonde hair: just pure chamomile tea, no oils after washing
for dark hair: rinse with henna but leave out the oils

Well-weighted and freely moving hair, cut in a style that allows your neck to be seen, and a loose scalp free from accumulated tension will not only enhance beauty. Looking after the hair and scalp will refresh and revitalize you, and liven up your mood.

CHAPTER SIX

The Forehead

The Extended Forehead

We tend to think of the forehead as the area between the eyebrows and the hairline. To turn the forehead into a feature that both looks and feels good, however, we need to extend the area beyond its ordinary limits. In movement and in the physical body nothing is defined by boundaries: everything is interconnected. In order to get the forehead working, think of it as a crossroads with one road going sideways above the eyes and below the temples, where the temporal muscles lie, and the other going upwards from the nose bridge, through the scalp, to the back of the neck. By feeling the temporal muscles working, you will be able to use them, together with the muscles on the scalp, to flatten out and tone up the forehead so that it will become a smooth, relaxed bed for positive thought and feeling.

Hiding the Forehead

Women frequently try to conceal a wrinkled neck with collars and scarves, and a lined and tense forehead with a fringe. This is as ridiculous as when a bald man grows the three hairs on one side of his head to cover the other half. When the wind blows, he is in trouble. Fashion offers many tricks. Unfortunately many of those tricks don't help at all in the long run. I see so many young girls and women wearing their hair in a way that can only encumber them; I sometimes wonder how they can see and move at all. One example was the girl who came to the studio complaining of migraine. She was also on antibiotics for an eye infection that wouldn't go away. I took one look at her hairstyle and understood the problem: her fringe was hanging fashionably low to one side, almost totally covering her right eye. She was holding her head at an angle that allowed her to see out of the remaining left eye. No wonder she had a stiff neck and eye infection! I explained the problem to her, gave her the "bench treatment" (see Chapter 11, Shoulders, Neck and Chin) and within a few days she was better.

Permanent off-balance carriage of the head causes neck cramps, which, when not relieved, can develop into chronic headaches. A fringe, picking up dust and dirt from the air and hanging into the eyes, might well have caused the eye infection. A long thick fringe is not only unhygienic, it also damages head posture and eyesight. In some men, forehead problems manifest themselves in a different way.

Protruding Eyebrow Syndrome

This is a feature which is noticeable in many powerful elderly men like politicians, businessmen and academics. A protruding eyebrow is swollen and sunken, with a hard layer of fat tissue and hardened muscle tissue stuck permanently between the eyebrows, causing a permanent expression of worry, anger and seriousness. Physiologically, the protruding eyebrow is actually a mixture of an overdeveloped muscle (from frowning) and an accumulation of stress and tension in that area.

The condition is usually accompanied by sinus, breathing and headache problems. Muscle tissue which is permanently contracted forms itself into tiny little knots or spasms, preventing free flow of fluids, air and electric force (energy). Mucus blocks the upper part of the nasal cavity and adds to the "traffic jam" of energy stuck in the area. Breathing and relaxation exercises and localized massage can help to unblock this junction of stuck forces.

The Temporal Muscles

The temporal muscles, lying just above the ears, are the main tool for toning up the face. Unfortunately, they are dormant in most people. The temporal muscle is a large shell-shaped muscle covering the hollow part above each ear. The following exercise will make you feel that the temporal muscle exists and that it can contract and tone up the entire face.

Ⓑ **Exercise No.29**   **Feeling the Temporal Muscles**

Put the hands flat on the temples, fingers resting on the scalp.

1. Start making chewing movements with the jaws closed.
   Do 25 to 30 repetitions of this movement while gently pressing the temples up and outwards.
2. Close your eyes, relax and breathe freely while faintly feeling the temporal muscles contracting and releasing under the palms of your hands, this time on their own, without moving the jaw.

Wrinkles

It is important to realize that you yourself are the one who has created your lines and wrinkles. The bulk of the work in wrinkle elimination consists of *not* doing rather than doing something about it. But that is also the hardest part: freeing yourself from old conditioned habits that cause your face to develop ageing wrinkles. Keep the nice wrinkles by all means, but get rid of the nasty ones. Before treating wrinkles, always make sure that the face is clean and cover the area with one of the following:

- glycerine
- petroleum jelly (Vaseline)
- a base oil (without any essential oils added to it)
- Nivea
- raw egg
- cream

Glycerine makes the skin feel warm and slippery; it is also a good rejuvenator as it is full of protein. It is a good idea to change what you use on your face every time you carry out these exercises. Let your own skin choose its preferences. Fig 34 shows you which lines enhance your expression and those that make you look most unfriendly.

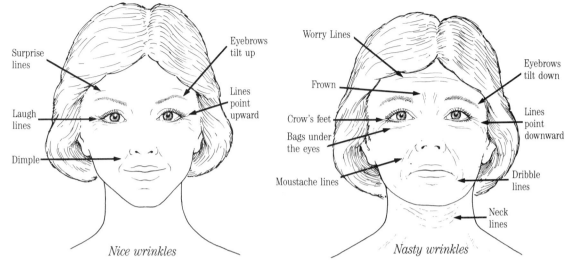

Fig 34: *Wrinkle map*

Ⓑ Exercise No.30

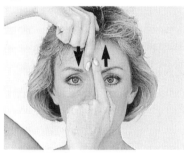

Fig 35: *Using two fingers in opposition across a wrinkle*

Ironing Out Wrinkles

Firstly make the surrounding area supple by applying oil, cream or whatever you are using on your skin. Work two index fingers in opposition to each other across the whole length of a wrinkle as illustrated here.

1. Move the fingers up and down in alternating fashion without scraping, pulling or stretching the skin but by moving the underlying muscle tissue over the bone structure without actually changing the position of the fingers on the skin.

   Do 15 to 20 repetitions of the movement along each line until you see the skin on either side of the wrinkle becoming a little red. That is when enough blood has been guided towards the area, preparing it for the next phase of wrinkle treatment.

Ⓘ Exercise No.31

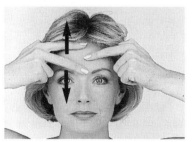

Fig 36: *Rubbing out wrinkles*

Rubbing Out Wrinkles

1. Hold two fingers on either side of the wrinkle. Gently open out the wrinkle with one finger of your other hand. Use your index finger, or if your nails are too long, use a knuckle. Now literally rub out the wrinkle as if you were using the rubber on the top of a pencil.
2. You will see that as you press harder, the skin immediately under the line changes colour from white, when the pressure is on it, to quite dark red when the blood is allowed to flow into the area. You will see the depth of the line diminishing as you work.
3. Don't rub for more than three or four times on each wrinkle in the beginning until your skin gets accustomed to being handled in this way.

Most importantly, remember never to iron out a wrinkle without first creaming the area with plenty of lubricant (see list above).

The Worry Line

Identify your worry line, if you have one, by looking at the wrinkle map in Fig 34 and look at the expression on your face. You may see the worry line emerging in the top centre part of the forehead.

(A) **Exercise No. 32**   ## Elimination of Worry Line

Put two fingers just above the worry line, with a gentle upward pull so that the line disappears.

1. While remaining in this position, contract the little muscles just under the worry line downward. Your hands are preventing the line from appearing.
2. Make up to 100 repetitions of this very small contraction against resistance, faster and stronger, releasing the hand hold to almost nothing until you feel that the muscles are getting very tired.
3. Hold this position for the same number of counts, then very slowly, still to the same beat, release the contraction until your forehead is relaxed again.

Be careful not to move any other part of the face or forehead while you are working and forget about worry and fear until you confront a worrying or fearful situation. Throughout the day, relax the forehead, face, neck and shoulders.

The Frown

The job of making a permanent frown disappear is not easy, but it is possible. Firstly you must loosen up the bundle of muscle that holds the frown in its place. If you died tomorrow your corpse would not show a frown; the spasmed muscles holding it would have finally let go — so why wait until then, when these exercises can help you get rid of it now?

Ⓑ Exercise No.33 — Ironing Out a Frown

Prepare the area with lots of glycerine, petroleum jelly or one of your favourite oil mixtures.

1. Gently massage the frown to loosen it.
2. Now place a finger on either side of the frown and pull ever so slightly to make the frown flat.
3. Hold this for eight counts while taking a deep breath.
4. Let go and see it shrinking back into its usual fold.
5. Now press hard against the flat frown and hold for eight counts, while at the same time pulling the muscles outward and upward.
6. Release the hold.
7. Finish by tapping the area with your fingertips as fast as you can until it feels warm and tingly.

Tell the little muscles between your eyebrows that you don't want them to contract. Tell them that you are not angry any more, that you don't need a frown. When you get angry that will be the right time to show a frown. Not right now, while you are trying to get rid of it. And don't, above all, get angry at not being able to get rid of your frown. It's going to be some weeks yet before your dormant muscles will obey you, but don't give up. Do this exercise every day until you see improvement.

Ⓘ Exercise No.34 — Frown Stretcher

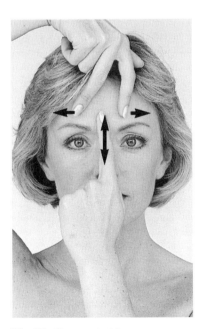

Fig 37: *Frown stretcher*

Now that you can feel the space between your eyebrows clear and empty, place three fingers on the side of your forehead as illustrated. The movement in the frown stretcher consists of lifting and expanding the arch of the eyebrows without making lines in any part of the forehead. Use the hands to guide the forehead upward and outward towards the hairline.

1. In this lifted position, begin to make small frowning movements against resistance. You can assist in the action with your eyes by focusing upwards and outwards.
2. A good number of little contractions to work up to is about 300 at fast speed, hold it for 50, then very slowly release over 50 counts. You will see that, for a brief moment, your forehead will remain in the large, stretched, newly toned position. Repeat this exercise daily and soon enough, it will stay like that permanently, provided of course that you stop tensing and wrinkling during the day.

Contraction against resistance encourages new muscle units to come out of hibernation from the depths of the frown lines under the skin. Exercising them, by immobilizing the muscle units that normally do the work, will divide the action evenly over the area which will become broader and freer. Eventually, the movement of frowning can be done imperceptibly, very finely, without visibly moving a muscle.

Frown Check

When you are typing, sewing, working or concentrating on any type of activity where you know you are likely to be frowning but can't help yourself doing it, just take a little piece of stiff gauze, put a little cream on the spot where the frown is and firmly stick the piece of gauze there. It will stick on to the cream, until you frown too heavily, when the gauze will fall off. This is an ideal way of checking the involuntary movements that you are making in the area. When the gauze falls off, just lick it, stick it back on and carry on with your work. If you work in a large office or factory you might get some funny looks when you do this, but if you work from home or in a place where people are sympathetic to self-improvement, they will smile and accept your eccentric behaviour.

Line Above the Eyebrows

The eyebrows are tricky in that on the one hand they are the main instrument for facial expression, and on the other the cause of much wrinkling in the forehead. The challenge is how to be expressive without being wrinkled, and also how to lift drooping eyebrows that hang downwards and make you look like a tired old dog. The following exercise involves the eyebrows' natural moves of lifting against hand resistance until the forehead is smooth and the brows become, once again, as youthfully expressive as in childhood.

Ⓐ Exercise No.35   Ironing the Forehead

Fix your hair up out of the way and apply cream to the forehead before starting. Lift the eyebrows once without holding the forehead and observe the lines created.

Put your hands on your forehead, fingers facing in and the "ball" of your hands resting on the temples. The grip is fairly firm with an upward and outward pull.

1. Now begin to lift your eyebrows and feel the movement under your fingers. Watch in the mirror and make sure no lines appear anywhere. You are lifting your eyebrows against the resistance of your hand. The muscles immediately underlying the lines are toning up and invigorating your skin.
2. Make the movement faster and faster, up to 500 times at more advanced stages. Hold your forehead firmly and don't allow it to wrinkle while you are working. The movements must become faster and smaller while the overall lift is increased. The muscles on your forehead should almost ache with exhaustion by the time you have finished.

3. Slowly diminish the pressure of your hands and slow down the contractions until you gradually take your hands off completely and cease moving. This may take a few sessions to perfect. Allow yourself to feel relaxation glowing all over your forehead while maintaining a flat, unlined surface with your eyebrows still slightly higher than they were before.

You will soon find that you will be able to raise an eyebrow without creating a wrinkle. The feeling at the end of this exercise is that you no longer have a forehead. If you don't wrinkle you should not be aware of your forehead, just as you don't usually feel your knee-cap. It's just there quietly resting in its place until needed.

Plaster Treatment

This rather extreme wrinkle treatment for the forehead should only be performed when circumstances in life leave you no choice and not more than once a fortnight. If, for example, you have not had your full quota of sleep and have an important luncheon date the following morning, or if you have been in very hot sunshine or have been concentrating too much and have a frown that you can't get rid of. Have one night's sleep with your forehead plastered up as illustrated below. The best type of plaster to use is ordinary fabric sticking plaster.

Make sure you sleep on your back for most of the night. If you tend to move a lot in your sleep this might prove difficult but propping yourself up with a couple of pillows will help you to move less. Two small cushions in the hollow part of the neck will stabilize the head. If the head is kept still the rest of the body is usually also quiet. Relax the face before you go to sleep, and sleep with the plaster on. In the morning keep the plaster on until you have your bath or shower. Gently soaking it with water will make removal painless and effortless. Do it patiently without ripping the plaster off. That would pull and severely stretch your skin. As the plaster comes off your forehead you will see a lovely smooth surface, like the skin of a baby. Your forehead could be like this all the time if you stopped frowning and wrinkling and twitching. Frequently check with your hands throughout the day that the forehead is relaxed.

Do this especially when you are carrying out tasks that are either demanding from a manual co-ordination aspect, or tasks that require you to concentrate mentally and visually as in sitting over a book, typewriter or a computer. Meanwhile keep observing other people's faces and their positive and negative facial habits to remind yourself to control your own.

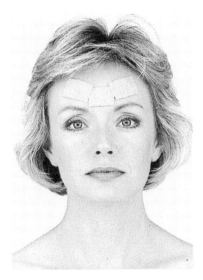

Fig 38: *Plaster treatment*

Caution — Tape, Skin and Blisters

Dancers often stick plaster all around the toes and heels to prevent the feet from hurting and blistering inside the point shoes. I remember that if the plaster wasn't taken off at night for more than one night, the skin under it would become all thick and white and just begin to peel off like a huge blister, leaving underneath a painful layer of bright pink raw flesh. It seemed that if the skin was deprived of air for more that 24 hours it would just die and fall off. Because the underlying flesh thinks that the tape is skin, it does not produce new skin. Instead it just remains raw flesh. Consequently when the plaster is ripped off after a day or two, you find raw flesh underneath. So please don't do to your forehead what we, stupid dancers, did to our feet.

Never use plasters on any part of the face but the forehead. The skin on the forehead is tight on the bone and cannot stretch easily. It is also the only part of the face that you don't need to move very much. If a plaster is applied on any other part of the face it will do more harm than good because it will a) stretch the skin too much when it is pulled off, and b) hinder movement.

Remember

You should make sure that you never feel your forehead tensing. But when you do feel a twitch, be aware of it and ask yourself where that twitch came from. Was it a reaction to something someone said? Was it a cringe against a sudden loud noise? Find out more about the external impulses that make your face move involuntarily, and try to eliminate uncalled-for movements.

CHAPTER SEVEN

The Eyes

You can't buy good posture in a shop, or a good facial expression in a supermarket. As usual, the essentials are free. Looking after yourself does not just mean keeping yourself clean and well dressed. Clothes are enhanced by good posture and style of movement. An expensive hair-do is wasted on an unbalanced head. The canvas for make-up is the quality of your skin, muscle tone and expression. The spark of your face is in the eyes. Not only is sight the sense most relied upon for effective functioning, but the eyes are also the window to the soul, conveying true inner feelings. This chapter will teach you how to expand your field of vision, improve your eyesight and at the same time rejuvenate the area surrounding the eyes to turn them into expressive and friendly gateways to your personality.

This is made possible by training the powerful ring muscle that holds your eye in its socket and teaching the little auxiliary muscles hidden behind it to obey your commands.

The Eyes as Receptors

As receptors the eyes should be broad enough to take in the maximum periphery while at the same time being able to focus on the smallest speck. The eyes can be selective about images that are bombarded at them. You don't have to watch the news or horror movies every day; there is plenty of horror in the streets. Stop and look when you meet a smiling child, coloured flowers or a sunset. Fill your "eye bank" with positive images and your vision will become more receptive to them. Let negativity influence what you see and you will forget to recognize beauty and fun.

The Eyes as Reflectors

As instruments of expression eyes should be clear, direct and a true reflection of how you feel at any given moment. Look at a child's eyes and see the openness, often called innocence. Physiologically, a young child's eyes are more open than an adult's eyes simply because gravity has not yet managed to pull down the surrounding area. A healthy adult eye can also be free of tense frowns, crow's feet and eye bags. Without cluttering up your expression, your eyes as reflectors show your true inner being. Do the exercises that follow step by step, but don't do more than two new exercises daily, as your body needs time to adjust to new moves.

Caution

The skin around the eyes is very thin and fragile. Before touching this delicate skin, it is very important to lubricate it with glycerine, petroleum jelly or sweet almond base oil. Never put any essential oils near the eyes. They are very strong and could sting or cause damage. If you need to touch your eyes and have no cream at hand, just lick your fingers and the saliva will temporarily protect the sensitive skin around the eyes from harm. Always begin working on your eyes by relaxing them to clean them from visual and nervous clutter and to make them fresh and ready to learn.

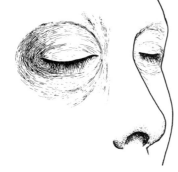

Fig 39: *The eye muscles*

Ⓑ Exercise No.36

Relaxing the Eyes

You will need:

- a dark room
- a flat surface to lie on
- some peace and quiet.

Lying flat on your back, pull up the knees and place the feet slightly apart, aiming for relaxed comfort. Close your eyes, cover them with the palms of your hands, and rest them in pure darkness for a few moments. Feel the little muscles of the eyelids pulsating.

1. Gently put both hands (palms down) on the closed eyes and relax. Listen to your own breath for a few minutes until you see nothing but

clean black behind the eyelids. If patterns and wild pictures appear at first, make them go away by telling your eyes that there isn't anything there for them to see. Tell your eyes to relax and accept total darkness. This might take a few minutes. Try to minimize and slow down the emerging images by reasoning with yourself that what you are seeing is left over imprints of what you saw when your eyes were open, but that at the moment your visual field should be empty of eye strain, pictures and light.

2. In this peaceful state, gently feel the shape of your eye sockets. Feel the small involuntary movements your eyes are making under your fingers.

3. Calm your eyes down so that they stop moving to achieve a neutral, relaxed state.

4. Take your hands away and allow your eyes to relax again deeply while breathing normally but consciously. Stay in this position with your eyes closed for as long as you like. Memorize the feeling of holding your eyes inside their sockets without any effort or tension.

Massage Technique No. 4

Eye Massage

Whenever your tired eyes need a rub, or if you get a piece of dirt in your eye, don't rub your fists violently into your eye sockets, thereby crinkling, squashing and folding your poor old skin until you see stars. Instead, give your eyes the following gentle eye massage to empty out bags and broaden your vision.

Before you start, remember to apply cream or oil to your face. Sweet almond base oil on its own will not sting.

1. Gently press the sides of your thumb against your upper eyelid and put your forefinger on the eyebrow. You can feel the edge of your eye socket. To become fully aware of the potential movement possibilities around the eye, trace around each eye socket gently with your fingers, just feeling their shape and size.

2. Now feel all the muscle tissue filling up the space between the bone of the eye socket and the underlying eyeball itself and ask the question: "How much of this flesh is active living matter (i.e. muscle) and how much of it is fat or flab?"

The following eye toning exercises will help to eliminate puffy eyelids, bags and crow's feet in less time than you thought possible.

Puffy Eyelids

Like bags, puffy eyelids are unsightly and hinder your sight. A puffed-up eyelid can be toned by making closed eye contractions against resistance.

Ⓑ Exercise No.37

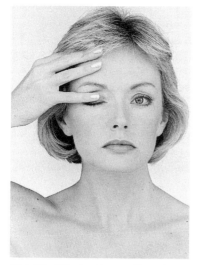

Fig 40: *Eliminating puffy eyelids*

Eliminating Puffy Eyelids

Place your hand on one side of your forehead, with two fingers resting on your brown bone. Place your little finger on your closed eyelid to feel its movement during the exercise, as illustrated in Fig 40.

1. Contract your upper eyelid firmly against the resistance of your finger. This contraction is not a squeeze or a squint. You are pulling your eyelid down towards your jaw bone, and inward, towards your eyeball. At the same time, raise your eyebrows. You can feel the movement happening under your little fingers.
2. When you feel the movement clearly and you are confident of doing it right without lifting or wrinkling your forehead, try to take your hands off gradually.
3. Contract and release 20 or more times, before feeling exhaustion in the muscles involved.
4. Finish the sequence by increasing the pressure on the inner and upper corner of the eye socket until you feel a not-too-uncomfortable pain (acupressure). Breathe through the pain deeply right down to the base of your abdomen and hold your breath for a while. Then breathe out slowly while releasing the pressure.

   Take your time over this.

The ideal shape to aim for is a slightly hollow upward curve which pushes the eyebrows up and out (think of Greta Garbo or Marlene Dietrich). It requires considerable application, at first, to keep everything under control but don't worry, it will become easier with practice.

Eye Bags

Eye bags make you look tired. Or do you get eye bags because you are tired? Lack of sleep, too much alcohol, smoking, water retention and obesity cause eye bags. A dirty or smoky atmosphere, forcing the eyes to stay half-closed for most of the time, does not help either. But if you have eye bags, the following toning exercise will help you lose the nasty things, or better, lose their contents, which is a mixture of dirty water and fat tissue and will, with exercise, be absorbed by the body and rejected through the normal excretion channels. If your bags persist, despite good sleep and exercise, try chopping an onion once or twice a week which will make you cry the debris out — but be careful never rub your eyes while handling onions.

Ⓑ Exercise No.38 — Eye Bag Removal

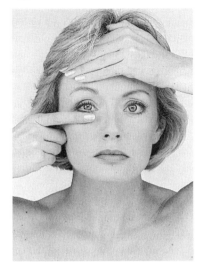

Fig 41: *Lower lid contraction*

Put your forefinger across the cheek bone as illustrated. Again, use only a gentle touch and make sure the skin is moist and slippery. Use the other hand throughout for control.

The exercise consists of the same action as in the previous exercise for external corner contractions, but you are now putting the emphasis in a different place. The muscles around the eye are ring muscles like those around the mouth or anus. However, when working on a specific area for a specific purpose, don't think of it as one large ring muscle, but direct your cerebral commands towards the particular part of the eye you are working on. For the number of repetitions and final procedure involving acupressure, breathing and relaxation, please refer to the previous exercise. The acupressure point here is on the bone under the eye bags, as shown on the acupressure map on page 13.

Eventually, both contraction exercises may be performed with your eyes closed whenever you find a spare moment. But wait until you have improved co-ordination and erased crow's feet before doing these with your eyes closed, as you will get more feeling and control initially by doing the exercises with your eyes wide open.

Crow's Feet

Ⓑ Exercise No.39 — Crow's Feet Extinction

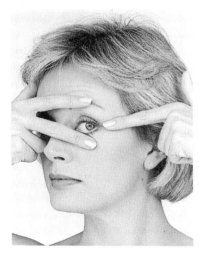

Fig 42: *Crow's feet extinction*

Crow's feet make you look as if it hurts you to laugh. With a little help from your fingers, they will soon go away.

The way to get rid of crow's feet is to perform external eye corner contractions against resistance. Lick your index finger and put it against the outer corner of your eye, making sure you gently flatten the lines. Use your other hand to keep everything else still.

1. Your eye is quite rightly going to react to the pressure of your finger on the outside corner and you will at first feel some twitching movements there.
2. As your eye gets used to the touch and understands that your fingers aren't going to poke it, you will be able to hold your finger in this position and keep your eye open, still and relaxed.
3. At this stage, you may start contracting your lower lid.
   Begin with eight repetitions for each eye. When you get better, double the number.

The movement you feel when doing a lower eyelid contraction is like a squint, but without the usual grimace that goes with a squint. Each contraction and release can be clearly felt under your index finger. Try to keep your eye open as wide as possible while contracting your lower lid. Be your own judge as to how many repetitions (between 20 and 50) are a good number for you. It is helpful to work to music that has a regular beat. Don't forget to count, as you are going to do the same number of repetitions with your other eye in a moment. Carry on until you feel your lower eyelid getting very tired but before you stop, increase the speed to double time and make the contractions smaller and smaller until there is no movement left, only a firmly toned muscle. Now tell the outside corner of your eye that this is its place, this is where it lives.

4. End with firm pressure against the acupressure point on the outer and upper corner of your eye socket (see acupressure map on page 13) with the usual breathing and slow relaxation procedure.

In a few weeks' time, as your co-ordination improves, your eyes will become clear and lively again, and your crow's feet will vanish.

Note: Beware of your forehead. Keep your forehead relaxed and check by feeling with your fingers that you are not frowning or lifting your eyebrows. Meanwhile, don't get into bad habits. Catch yourself laughing and keep your eyes more open as you laugh.

Your Visual Periphery

Your visual periphery is how far you can see around you. The bigger and clearer your eyes, the more they will let you see. So lift the heavy curtains of drooping eyelids and swollen bags, and you will enjoy wider vision. Tiny little angry and suspicious-looking eyes are not going to make you look very good. If your drooping eyelids cover any part of the iris when you look straight ahead, then your eyes are lazy and we shall wake them up by expanding your periphery.

Ⓑ **Exercise No. 40**   **Expanding the Periphery**

Place your fingers against your forehead and your thumbs on your cheekbones, gently pressing upward as shown.

1. Observe the periphery of your visual field. How far can you see around by moving your eyeballs only? Starting at 12 o'clock (straight upwards), slowly work your gaze around the clock. Notice how certain areas, like perhaps one o'clock, are overshadowed by a dropped brow. Or you may meet the top of a cheek when looking down to eight o'clock. Go round

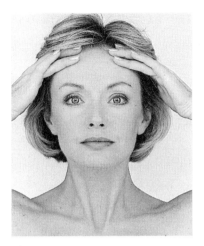

Fig 43: *Expanding the periphery*

both ways slowly, noticing the boundaries at every hour. When you have clearly defined the shape and size of your periphery you can begin expanding it with gentle help from your hands.

2. Place your hands on either side of your forehead so that they are just out of sight, gently lifting any shadows out of the way. Now do the clock exercise again slowly both ways. You will now see that the circumference of your periphery is completely clear and much bigger. Should you feel any tension at the back of your neck at this stage, stop and go back to the relaxation exercise for a minute or two. When your eyes are rested repeat the exercise once more. This time use less help from your hands; make the muscles work instead. Eventually, if you do this exercise frequently you will be able to keep your field of vision broad and clear with no help from your hands at all. When you are good at expanding the periphery you will enjoy doing it at any time, in any permissible situation. Of course, if you do it incorrectly and start twitching your eyebrows at the dinner table for no apparent reason, you might have some explaining to do.

Expanding the periphery is the most beautiful exercise in the whole of this book. It will lift your mood on a grey day, or any time you feel like being happy. Expanding the periphery will make your eyes bigger and give you a fresh view of the world.

Better Eyesight

It goes without saying that for eyes to look good, they must also function well. Visual impairment can be treated with exercises. When you notice the first signs of eye weakness or unevenness, begin doing some of the following exercises and you will never need to wear glasses. If you are already wearing glasses or contact lenses, wear them less frequently and try the exercises. You will soon find that your eyes will need a weaker correction lens. Glasses or lenses are to bad eyesight what crutches are to a cripple. Crutches can help a cripple get around but they will not cure the lameness. Only therapeutic exercise can improve or cure bad eyesight. Glasses prevent free spontaneous movement of your head; they make your eyes lazy. Contact lenses are perhaps less cumbersome, but a piece of plastic stuck to an eyeball cannot really be comfortable, however much the friendly body is prepared to adapt. Unless irreparable damage has taken place and sight is totally inadequate, glasses and lenses should not be worn. For the severely visually impaired, the exercises given here will be of great benefit. Even if the exercises may not cure the most severe visual handicaps, they will give improvement and help to retard or arrest further deterioration. For people who have no need for glasses, the exercises will ensure that it will stay that way.

Balancing the Eyes

Sitting in a relaxed position, holding this book, put your left hand on to your closed left eye and just carry on reading. Notice if there is any difference between reading with one eye, the other eye or both. Find out if one eye is weaker than the other and if this is so continue reading with your weak eye until it becomes uncomfortable. You may find that it will become easier after it gets worse, so persevere for a little while. Most people have a weaker eye; it's perfectly normal, as they say. Perfectly normal doesn't mean it is all right. A weak eye is like a visual limp. It means that your strong eye is overloaded with work, getting exhausted while your weak eye, relying on your strong eye, is getting lazier and weaker all the time. Eyes are living organisms that can change and improve. Improvement is often instant, as you will find out when you work through the focusing exercises. Are you still reading with your weak eye? If not, go back a few lines.

Ⓑ Exercise No. 41

Focusing

There are two dots printed next to each other on the next line.

•   •

Focus on the dot on the right while being aware that the other dot is there, but appears blurred. Now reverse: look at the left dot with the right one unsharp, out of focus. Repeat changing your focus from one dot to the other, doing it faster and faster. The quicker the eyes are able to change focus, the sharper they will be. Now try the same thing with the dots closer together:

•   •

and closer still:

• •

This simple focusing exercise can be done anywhere, at any time with any two or more focal spots. Experiment with spots on posters in the bus or the underground, or on two moving leaves on a tree. With a little imagination, any background can serve as a focal exercise field. You can play around by changing the distance between your focal spots.

Text focusing — reading

Try reading the following sentences printed here in different point sizes.

This line is printed in 12 point and is very easy to read.

Different words printed in 10 point are a bit smaller but still no problem to read.

This book is not printed in 8 point because some people would have trouble reading it.

As for 6 point print, that must be for people who eat a lot of carrots.

4 point print is readable only to those with ultra-clear vision.

Experiment with reading the above lines with both eyes together, then with one eye at a time and find out at which point size, if any, your eyes become weak. Read the difficult line again with the strong eye. Memorize not the content of the sentence but the shapes of the letters as you are reading with the better eye. Now try again reading the same sentence with the bad eye. The memory obtained of the image with the strong eye will help the weak eye decipher the blur. You may not believe your own eye, but the weak eye learns to focus as sharply as the strong eye in this way. When you get to a line that is not readable even with the strong eye, get a magnifying glass and look at the shape of the letters. Put the magnifying glass away and recall the meaning of the words to help you memorize and visualize the shapes of the letters. Now try reading the line again without the magnifying glass. The shapes of the letters in very small type will emerge. Repeat this until you get results, but only to a level of acceptable tolerance. As soon as you feel your eyes getting tired, cover them with the palm of your hands and relax to complete the exercise.

Depth focus — zoom

Standing by the window chose a spot or mark on the window pane and focus upon it. Now without moving the head find a focal point directly behind that mark, some object or point far away outside the window. As in the previous exercise, the object here is to focus alternately between the two chosen spots, while maintaining an awareness of the other spot as an unsharp object that is ready to be focused upon. If you are sure that you have a weaker eye, your eyesight can be improved in this way without spending any extra time. While you are at home alone or with your family, cover up the strong eye with a pad and carry on with normal activities. This will train the weak eye to catch up a bit and give the overworked eye a good rest. Of course, if visitors arrive, make sure you take the pad off or they will wonder what's wrong with you.

The Sun: Is it Good or Bad for You?

How much light can your eyes tolerate? The eyes, being just as user-friendly as the rest of your body, have a wide tolerance for light or the lack of it, but with limitations as always. Long, dark, winters with no sunshine for weeks on end, make your eyes less tolerant to bright light. When suddenly the sun comes out, even a mere bleak, cloudy shimmer of a sun, people in the streets squint and rush out to buy sunglasses. It is not uncommon for people living in big cities to get up before the sun, travel on the underground to an artificially-lit workplace and return home at night after the sun has set. This means that, for several months, many people don't see the sun or any daylight at all, apart from at weekends if they bother to leave the house . . . no wonder they squint on the first sunny morning like prisoners just released from dark chambers. Depression, the winter blues (or SAD — Seasonal Affective Disorder), and many ailments and psychological disorders can be attributed to light deprivation. Light is life. Plants live on light, air and water. Humans, who need so many things to live often forget the basics like light and air. So, contrary to Californian advice to avoid bright sunshine, if you live in a climate where sunshine is scarce, I recommend you feed your eyes with natural light whenever you get a chance.

(A) Exercise No.42   Sun Focusing with Care

Note: There is a lot of scared talk at the moment about the dangers of the sun, the broken ozone layer and skin cancer from exposure to sunlight. As mentioned above, if you live in a hot, dry climate where the sun is shining all the time, then avoid the sun. Too much of a good thing will harm you. These sun focusing exercises should only be carried out during the winter months, preferably when the sky is semi-cloudy and when the sun appears weak and pale. In addition, they should never be performed in the middle of the day when the sun is at its highest. The best time to do these is at sunrise or sunset, when the sun is far enough away not to burn at all.

Stand in a park or garden somewhere outdoors as far away from traffic and pollution as possible, and palm the right eye (see page 102).

1. Peering through the gaps between your fingers, find the sun hiding behind a white cloud or a tree and focus upon it. Keep looking at the distant sun until it stops wobbling around and you see a perfect white circle. At this point, breathe in deeply. Your solar plexus will jump and you should experience a sudden feeling of ecstasy.
2. Now palm both eyes and relax them. The imprint of the sun on your retina is not really there; make it go away as soon as possible, and see pure, clean darkness.
3. When you are rested from the experience, repeat sun focusing with your left eye and again relax both eyes.
4. As soon as your eyes are able to see pure black again, slowly open them and repeat with both eyes together.

Do this exercise only once a week in the beginning, until you feel you would like to do it more often (weather permitting).

You may not be able to do all three exercises straight away. Tears might start pouring out of your eye in the beginning. This is nothing to worry about; use the tears to wash the affected eye and try again next time. It might take quite a while before you are able to do the last exercise — looking at a pale sun with both eyes simultaneously. Use your hands to shade your eyes if the light is too bright at first. Just peep through your fingers if you can't take it.

The advantages of feeding your eyes with sunlight are that they will become sharper, brighter, more shiny, younger looking and more efficient. As a long distance focusing exercise to improve depth of vision, nothing can beat sun focusing. As a therapeutic exercise it works wonders: after a dull stretch of grey, drizzly weather, you can be guaranteed that careful sun focusing will lift your mood.

Going to Sleep

It is during sleep that your face can really relax and process all the new movement patterns you have been teaching it so far, but although there is something called "beauty sleep", which will be explained in a moment, sleeping can, in certain circumstances, badly damage your face. Every individual has a particular bedtime scenario. I wouldn't want to change your sacred bedtime routine if I can help it, just give you plenty of food for sleep. Each to their own, as they say.

In the Western world, it is considered good form to have a special room for sleeping. A pleasant room, with attractive furniture scientifically designed for the best possible night of sleep. So why do so many people suffer from insomnia? There is no room here to write a whole book on sleep. In the context of the face, sleep needs four vital things: comfort, silence, darkness and clean air. I have never found these in any sleeping pills. In addition to comfort, silence, darkness and fresh air you need to be tired both in body and spirit if you expect to go to sleep. If you've been doing inactive desk work all day, your brain will be tired but your body won't. How can your brain go to sleep if your body is wide awake? You'd better go for a jog around the block, then try sleeping again.

Silence — Relaxing the Ears

The ears are, like the eyes, receptors for stimuli. The ears feed sound messages to the brain, which classifies the messages into various departments. The ears, like any other part of the body, need rest. If the ears are constantly bombarded with noise, loud, soft or irritating, they will develop resistance to those noises. You no longer hear these irritants, causing permanent ear strain. Nevertheless, somewhere in your brain "computer" there is a chamber full of stored irritants in the form of these accumulated noises. If the situation is such that these irritants are constant they will eventually drive you crazy and stop you sleeping. In fact, insomniacs are in a way addicted to disturbances. Most insomniacs cannot go to sleep without a book, the television or sex. If they are left in their own company, they spend half the night thinking and puzzling instead of voluntarily giving their bodies over to rest.

Sleep is a funny thing. It will come automatically when you are tired both in body and mind. There is nothing as annoying as just lying there, waiting for sleep to be kind enough to arrive. Waiting is one of the most boring and frustrating states of being. Boredom is the most tiring form of occupation. Boredom occurs during dead time, waiting time. It will become more and more apparent to you while working through this book that you can arrange your life in such a way that you are never bored, and never have to waste your time. You can build up a stock of minimal and mental exercises which you can call upon at any dead bit of time. So whenever you are waiting patiently for something or someone (including sleep), don't fill up that time with negative thoughts. Bad thoughts are often a manifestation of discontentment or imbalance in the body. By using dead time with productive mental and physical exercise, you will exhaust both the mind and the body in a sleep-inducing way.

Degrees of Darkness

Light stimulation from sources such as left-on TV sets, or flashing green lights on video recorders, is as harmful for the eyes as irritating background noises are for the ears. To see how thin and translucent the skin of an eyelid is, do the following exercise at night-time. Playing with degrees of darkness has the benefit of relaxing the eyes while sharpening up focus. It will also improve your sense of balance and your confidence.

Ⓘ Exercise No.43

Focusing in the Dark

Sit on a chair in a dark room and close your eyes. You see darkness, or think you see darkness.

1. Put the palms of your hands on your eyes and see how much darker it has become.
2. Open your eyes. Are the curtains drawn? How much can you see in a dark room?
3. Switch the light on and memorize the shape of the objects in the room.
4. Turn the light off again and find the objects in the dark. How long does it take you to find your sight after switching off the light?

Repeat switching the light on and off and notice the speed at which you are able to readjust your focus.

Don't be scared of the dark. Explore it. Walk about in the dark room and see how the reduced light has affected the balance in your legs. This shows that we rely most heavily on visual orientation to stay balanced and not knock against things. If balance can be trained in darkness, this will relieve the eyes from energy they can spend on looking, rather than just seeing things.

Sleeping Positions

The body moves around through many different positions during a night's sleep. The movements are not random. Postural change during sleep is specifically programmed to rebalance your body after its daily activities. It is useful to analyse some of your postural habits during sleep and figure out why they are as they are. The following true tale will clearly illustrate this point.

I remember from my dancing days a particular occasion when we were rehearsing a modern dance passage containing numerous turns: a long combination of multiple turns, turns alone, turns with partner, fast ones, slow ones and so on. The awkward thing was that all these turns went in one direction: they all went clockwise. The rehearsal must have lasted about three hours, until late in the evening. I went to bed that night quite exhausted and fell asleep as soon as I lay down. During the night I became faintly aware of constantly rolling over and over. I woke up the next morning covered in sweat with all the sheets and covers wound around my body like a mummy. Interestingly, the direction of the drapings proved that my body had been rotating anti-clockwise! My user-friendly body had been untwisting all those clockwise turns I had been making during the rehearsal in an attempt to rebalance me.

Look at your face each morning when you wake up and see to what degree it has been folded into creases. By adopting a standard sleeping position before falling asleep, you can train your body to behave a little better at night.

Ⓑ Exercise No.44   Sleeping Position

It is impossible to control totally the movements made during sleep but what you *can* do is to adopt a standard position for going to sleep through relaxation.

The position that will least damage your face during sleep is lying on your back, with your head resting between two small pillows that are placed in the nape of the neck just to stop your head rolling off to the side. Large pillows are not recommended.

If you go to sleep every night in the above recommended position, your body, as it gets better balanced during the day, will move and twist less in sleep. Your face will get used to being held facing up and in this way creasing and folding during the night will be greatly reduced. Going to

Fig 44: *Sleeping position*

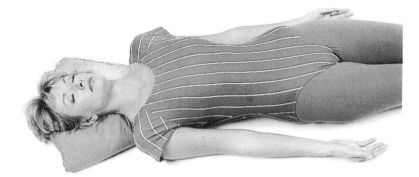

sleep can be a pleasant, conscious act instead of simply zonking out. You will find that the quality of your sleep will improve and that you will need a lot less sleep if you follow these brief guidelines.

Good Sleep Factors

- Have a cleaned massaged face.
- Check noise, light and air flow.
- No tight clothing, no elastic or buttons, preferably naked in cotton sheets.
- Use two small pillows.
- Perform the full facial relaxation as described in Chapter 2.
- Perform the eye relaxation exercise as shown on page 102-3.

If you are not asleep by now it means you don't need any sleep.

Get up and about; do something useful in the house that you have been putting off for weeks. If you can't find anything to do, go back to Chapter 1, Self-image, and do some postural correction exercises or practise the latest facial exercise you have learned in this book. Don't spend time thinking about your life and your situation. Occupy your mind with something of the here and now. It won't harm you at all, even if you spend the entire night on such activities. You won't feel particularly tired tomorrow and you will have enjoyed the silence of the night and the waking up of the birds. Your nocturnal experience will be yours and yours alone. With the help of the regeneration exercise described on page 43 you will soon pick yourself up if you feel weak tomorrow. It is possible to regenerate oneself more effectively from conscious relaxation and regeneration exercise than from a bad night's sleep in a stuffy, centrally heated, noise-humming room. The most important thing about insomnia is that it is not an illness, only a temporary state of being which can be changed with good practices and understanding. The statement "I suffer from insomnia" is nonsense.

You may suffer from tension, an unbalanced mind/body relationship, lack of creative output, an overfilled stomach and many other things, but "insomnia" is a sum total of other ailments which cannot be dozed off with tranquillizers. After a good night's sleep, waking up in the morning should be the most beautiful experience of each day of your life. Life is precious and short. A new day is another chance to see a sunset or a horizon, another chance to produce something of value to others. You are more important than any problem. Be equipped to enjoy this day, and to contribute towards making it a good day for those around you. Live your life, fully aware of your user-friendly body, your real self, and apply yourself positively to your daily activities.

CHAPTER EIGHT

The Cheeks

The cheeks are the largest part of the face. Almost like two flat sheets stretched across from the jaw to the temples and sideways towards the nose and the ears, the cheeks immediately reveal your facial tone. Ageing people lose the fullness of youth when the cheeks begin to sag, become hollow and fold down on to the jaw. Your cheeks may not yet have reached that stage, but I assure you they will eventually hang like empty bags if you don't begin toning them up right now. Being able to feel the difference between a relaxed cheek or a tight cheek is one of the most difficult things to learn, but once you have felt your cheeks contracting and releasing, you will be able to tone them in no time at all.

Sagging Cheeks

In both men and women (and dogs) the first signs of ageing manifest themselves in a break in the continuity of the jaw line. To understand the phenomenon of ugly sagging cheeks fully we should consider the purpose of having cheeks in the first place. The question is: are cheeks muscle groups to aid the chewing of food, or are they food storage units or bags as they are in the hamster or chipmunk?

Both diet and the way we eat affect the facial movement we perform with our cheeks. If the amount of food you put into your mouth is larger than the space provided for it (the cavity between the closed jaws) some of the food will be stored in the cheeks, at the side of the jaw. Many people happily eat like this. They put as much food in their mouth as it can hold, forgetting that the teeth need space to chew. About two-thirds of a large mouthful is stored in the cheeks. This will stretch the cheek, causing it eventually to become a bag when it is empty. A better way of eating is to take a bite only as big as your teeth can immediately cope with. Chew, swallow and empty your mouth before the next bite is put in. Although such basic table manners are taught to most civilized children, a look around restaurants might make you wonder.

Eating Observations

I suggest that one day, when you are on your own, you sit down in front of a large mirror and watch yourself eat. Notice all the movements your cheeks, jaws and mouth are making. Consider which of the movements are nice to look at and which are ugly. Is there a bit of food stuck in one of the holes in your teeth? Do you find yourself sometimes vigorously pulling down one mouth corner because your tongue is trying to retrieve some food lost in the cheek bags? As a rule, keep most of the food within the boundaries of your teeth. Anything falling outside of that area, even though still contained in your mouth, is too much to handle right now. Keep the food nicely together within the cavity of your closed jaws. Chew the food until you can swallow it easily without having to resort to a drink. Any mouthful of food should have 60 to 70 per cent of raw foodstuff in the form of vegetable, salad or fruit in it to moisten the remaining carbohydrates (bread, rice, pasta or any other "bulk"). This makes for easy swallowing once the food is all mixed up and chewed. The juices contained in the raw vegetables, mixed with your saliva and its digestive enzymes, are a healthier lubricant than a cold gulp of wine, beer or even pure water. If the diet is well-balanced, a drink at the table is not really necessary. Food should contain enough moisture from the juices within it. If you chew it well, you don't need to swallow any additional fluids. Save your drink until after the meal.

So remember, take smaller mouthfuls of food so you can move your face gracefully when eating. As soon as a bulge of food can be seen hidden inside the cheeks, it distorts the shape of the face and will turn you into a caricature of yourself. Over time your hamster-like eating habits will show in sagging cheeks.

Swallowing

When you swallow, don't retract your jaw but keep your teeth in the "cross" position described in Chapter 10, Mouth and Jaw. That is, the position whereby the two top front teeth are placed in line with the two bottom centre teeth. Constantly swallowing food down with a jaw retraction creates ugly lines above the chin and at the down side of the mouth corners. For movement and placement of the jaw, please refer to Chapter 10.

Toning the Cheeks

(B) Exercise No.45   Cheek Relaxation

Lie down flat on your back with the knees pulled up and relax. If your cheeks were drapes pinned on to your facial skeleton with drawing pins, there would be four pins in all: one on the external side of the temple, another pin just below the inner eye corners, a third on the lower corner of the jawbone, and the fourth pin would be at a point slightly above the upper lip as illustrated in Fig 45.

Remember these four points as important cities on the map of your facial landscape. Just quietly lie there and memorize each point in turn to train your consciousness to be aware of them. This conditions the area between the points to be more correctly placed and prepares you for the relaxation and toning exercises that follow.

1. Tilt your head to the right side so that it is resting peacefully. The left cheekbone should be the uppermost point.
2. Concentrating your mind on this highest point, imagine that your cheek is a soft sand dune and that the skin that covers it is very fine sand slowly rolling down in a warm summer wind. Gently relax the cheek and let its movement flow down towards its base.
3. As you do this, take in a deep breath, hold it for 10 counts and breathe out slowly.
4. Now roll your head gently from side to side, remembering how your cheek feels when it is relaxed, and compare that cheek with the other.
5. Turn your head towards the left side and repeat the relaxation for the right cheek.

Give special attention to the area nearest the corners of your mouth and make sure you are not biting the inside of your cheek or holding your tongue tight. While you are resting in this position notice how the other cheek, the one nearest to the floor, is beginning to hang downwards like an empty bag. When you are good at doing this relaxation exercise, you may proceed to isolating each cheek and toning them.

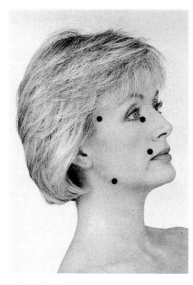

Fig 45: *The cheek support points*

118

ⓘ Exercise No.46   Cheek Isolation

Remain in the same relaxed position, the head tilted towards the left. Relax the neck and shoulder muscles.

1. You are going to divide your attention between the two cheeks. Keep your left cheek relaxed while gently contracting the right one so as to lift the part that is hanging down.

   If you have trouble contracting your cheek, imagine you are chewing the inside of your cheek, but without actually doing the action. The feeling is similar, but much, much smaller. If your cheeks are clearly hanging down in this position, the contraction may be felt more clearly. Use a hand to skim the contracting cheek in support of its effort and feel the cheek lifting up, getting harder and firmer under the palm of your hand.

   Do as many contractions as you can until a point is reached when you get tired; this may be between 30 or 50.

2. When your muscles feel tired, breathe more deeply. This will give you energy to do a few more.

3. End the sequence by speeding up the contractions until they become so small and so fast that the cheek seems to want to remain in this hovering state.

4. Repeat on the other side the same number of times unless you feel that one side needs more work. Don't forget to breathe and relax before you change over.

Be careful to isolate both cheeks, keeping one completely relaxed while working on the other.

It is this hovering state kept immobile which will give you the muscle tone you aspire to.

Ⓐ Exercise No.47   Cheek Contraction

The cheek contraction is similar in feeling to the previous exercise but stronger. You may do this exercise either lying down, standing up, or upside down looking through the legs. Each position will work the muscles in a different way and you should alternate between all available positions. By doing these in several different positions, your cheeks will develop muscle tone faster than if you were to stick to the same position all the time. Changing the position also gives more variety to the rest of your body while exercising, which makes it more interesting for you.

The cheek contraction involves contracting your entire cheek towards the four points shown in Fig 48. Take the contraction step by step, in eight counts.

1. Hold it for eight.
2. Release for eight.
3. Relax and breathe.

To get the right feeling, imagine an invisible force pulling your cheek towards each of the four points. Place a finger on each of the points as shown on the illustration, using both hands. Don't press your fingers into the skin, just hold them there to remind you where the action should be directed towards.

4. Repeat on the other side. When you are good at this you may do both cheeks at the same time without hand support. When you have begun to feel the muscles in your cheeks tightening you may go on to the next exercise which will make them stronger.

Ⓑ Exercise No.48

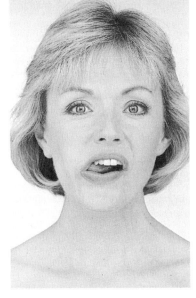

Fig 46: *Tongue in cheek*

Tongue in Cheek

Stand in front of a full-length mirror and formulate the shape of a large letter "O" with your mouth, making sure that the top lip is not wrinkled. While retaining this shape try to manage a smile, gently lifting the corners of your mouth.

1. Stick your tongue firmly against the inside of your right cheek. Don't forget to keep the rest of your face well relaxed.
2. Press against different parts of your inner cheek with the tongue by contracting the tongue as hard as it will go and pressing it firmly against the resisting inner wall of your cheek.
3. Make about 20 cheek contractions over the tongue on each side, frequently changing the position of the tongue under the cheek to reach all its parts.

Your tongue is acting as a pressure point inside the cheek which you should press firmly towards the tongue.

Apart from serving as a convenient pad for toning the cheeks, using the tongue has an additional beneficial side-effect. Its base, situated under the chin, is being pulled upward, thereby toning any double (or triple) chins you might have. The tongue in cheek exercise tones many different small muscle groups which will eventually harmonize together to give your cheeks, once again, a firm, youthful and healthy look.

Ⓘ Exercise No.49

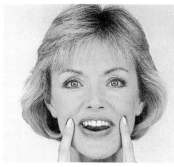

Fig 47: *Cheek dimpler*

Cheek Dimpler

One of the most effective exercises to tone up sagging or hollow cheeks which so unattractively breaks the jaw line is the cheek dimpler.

1. Make the large "O" shape with your mouth, smile and say the sound "RRRRR".
2. While continuing to make the sound, contract the lower front parts of your cheeks so that they move upwards and inwards towards the inside of your open mouth.
3. Gently place two fingers on these areas as illustrated in Fig 47 and feel the contraction working.
4. Make about 50 such small contractions or more until you feel the muscles immediately underlying your two fingers getting very tired.

5. Take a deep breath, move your jaw from side to side, relax and start again.

Repeat the whole exercise three times. I am giving you a heavy dose of the feeling in this part of the cheek to make you aware that this is *the* most important part to work on if you want to avoid looking like a saggy old bag. When you are aware of the feeling in this part of the cheek you may proceed with the next exercise.

Ⓐ **Exercise No.50**

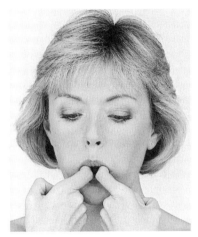

Fig 48: *Dimpler with resistance*

Dimpler with Resistance

Place an index finger on each inside of the cheeks, opposite the bottom teeth, in the same spot where your fingers were in the previous exercise but this time inside your mouth.

Perform the same contractions as in the previous exercise, this time pushing your cheek muscles firmly against the resisting finger on the inside. You can control the amount of effort you exert with your fingers. You can do it lightly, or harder, any way you choose.

Find a regular rhythm pattern and make between 20 and 30 repetitions, which will increase to 80 or 100 at more advanced stages.

You will find, at the end of the sequence, that the muscles in your lower cheeks will ache and feel slightly numb. This is very good for toning. You can get rid of the pain immediately after the exercise by releasing the muscles affected, shaking your head about, deep breathing and gentle massage. It is quite likely that these muscles will feel sensitive tomorrow; muscles always do when they have just been woken up. The best remedy for any stiffness there tomorrow is to repeat the exercise again.

Feeding Your Cheeks

As I have already mentioned, we know that the skin likes to be fed different things at different times. The cheeks, being the largest area on the face, need most feeding. If one day you wake up feeling rather groggy, with pale, dry cheeks from central heating, air conditioning or the heat outside, and if when walking towards the bathroom your first smile seems more like a grimace, why not treat your cheeks to breakfast? The list of natural nutrients that the face likes is endless. Some of the vegetable and dairy products that may be used are listed in Chapter 4, Clean and Feed, but you may very well discover new tastes by experimenting further for yourself. When your face is dry, use a dairy product or honey rather than vegetable or fruit juice. Feeding the face should be done at least once a week or whenever your face feels dry, stiff or sunburned. The nature of the food product is best chosen intuitively. Immediately after getting up, before you even have a chance to wake up fully, just ask yourself: "Does my face need anything, and if so, what?". You will get a response to which you should adhere without questioning why this particular foodstuff came to your mind (unless of course it is something so crazy that you know it might poison, endanger or hurt you).

Choose any ingredient given on the list. Most ordinary foods in the kitchen are quite safe.

The nutrient should be laid upon the warm and moist skin with its open pores ready to receive. It should be left on no longer than until it is almost dry; you may massage your face with it where it is itchy or where you feel a need for it. Never leave it on until it begins to crackle.

After feeding, wash off with almost cold water. Let your face dry naturally, and just before it is completely dry tap a small amount of sweet almond base oil on if it still feels stiff. If your face feels OK, just leave it naked and stay in a clean, airy and slightly moist environment.

(I) Exercise No.51   Cheek Tapping

Cheek tapping may be done daily after applying cream or while feeding the face.

Tap your cheeks all over with the pads of your fingers, while inflating them with air, for about 50 counts until they begin to tingle. Sense how certain parts seem firm, while others bits hang loose and flabby. Aim the tapping movements at the areas that have no bone underneath, and feel the muscles tightening under your fingers.

Tapping the cheeks will tone them up and stop them sagging. Tapping is also the best method for helping your skin absorb food or lubricant.

Facial Herb Sauna

When you have a cold or feel as if your skin is full of impurities, boil up a pan with your favourite herbs. I sometimes put in camomile, thyme, rosemary, dill, sage, or whatever I can lay my hands on in the herb garden or the kitchen. Adding fresh garlic to the concoction may seem smelly, but garlic is one of the best cleansing plants: its sharpness attacks bacteria and heals infections. Put the whole lot in a small amount of water in a (non-aluminium) pan and boil it up. When it has boiled for ten minutes or so sit at the table with a big towel over your head and allow the pores of your skin to breathe in the scented vapour. As you inhale all the differet smells, imagine where they came from: the fields, prairies, gardens . . . Imagine the landscape, the sky, the clouds, the wind and everything else that belongs to growth, warmth, and health. All the impurities in your skin and lungs will come out. Gently bathe your face in lukewarm water to wash off the dirt and splash with cold water to finish.

Hailstorm Massage

Once, we were walking across a hillside in Wales when a heavy hailstorm descended upon us. We were quite warm from walking, and the only choice seemed to be to continue as no shelter was available for miles around in this treeless landscape. This was initially unpleasant. Who wants to walk in a hailstorm? But as the rhythm of our pace harmonized with the elements, I began to feel great pleasure in the gentle tingling of my cheeks against the small grains of ice that hit them. On our return, sitting cosily by the warm wood fire, it felt as if my face had been exposed to a holiday at the seaside. I felt glowing, happy and healthy. At home you can simulate the Welsh hailstorm by splashing iced water on to your face as a final rinse after massage. Never touch your skin with actual ice as this will damage it. The ice-cold water will tighten the pores and make you look glowingly fit and young, and it is also an excellent measure against little red veins on the cheeks.

The amount, degree and frequency of exposure of this kind upon your face is entirely up to you, but the more it is exposed to the most varying types of stimuli the more alive it will be, provided that: 1) you are in control over what is happening and 2) any feeling from any action is pleasurable. It is evident from this that you should not expose the face to prolonged hot sun as that is most unpleasurable and hence very harmful to the skin.

① Exercise No.52

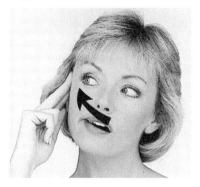

Fig 49: *Side cheek lift*

Side Cheek Lift

Make a small "O" with the mouth with the usual slight turn up of the corners of your mouth.

1. Move your whole mouth upwards towards the right temple as illustrated.
2. Focus your eyes into the same direction (roughly at one o'clock). Now you will notice on the side that is being pulled up that you have created some lines around the lifted mouth corner.
3. Using your hand, gently guide the wrinkles upwards so that they smooth themselves out. Tilt your temple upwards, towards the same diagonal direction.
4. With less and less help from the hands, teach your cheek muscles to hold the position all by themselves without creating any lines.

Try, at the same time as you are eliminating the lines, to reduce the aid that your hands are giving so that the cheek is performing the upward pull all by itself with the minimum amount of lines created. You can do this to music — chose any rhythm you like — and repeat the upward-pulling cheek and temple contraction 20 times or more, until the muscles feel tired.

End the sequence with breathing and relaxation before you attempt to do the other side.

Cheek Shakes

Occasionally, when you are very tense, you will feel like doing a cheek shake. They are not to be done too frequently or they would sag further the passive areas on your face. And unless you do this in the horizontal or upside-down position, so that your cheeks hang backwards and upwards, shaking will loosen them even further. It is best to do the upright cheek shake just once to feel how very loose and relaxed the cheeks can be.

Cheek shakes are very good for loosening those tight expressions in your face that create permanent wrinkles. If you are a lower tension carrier (see Chapter 3) you will benefit especially from cheek shakes. In addition, they are very good for people with fat cheeks.

Ⓑ Exercise No. 53 — Upright Cheek Shake

Stand firmly in the correct upright posture, feet slightly apart, knees relaxed, hips tucked under the spine, neck erect and the shoulders loose.

1. Slowly drop your head forwards. You may slightly curve your back if that is more comfortable.
2. Begin shaking your head from side to side, increasing the speed of its motion. You may produce a sound while doing this. Sound with movement helps to release tension and cleans the channels that carry energy flow.

Ⓘ Exercise No. 54 — Horizontal Cheek Shake

Lying flat on your back, shake your head, which is resting on the floor, gently from side to side. Make sure all the flesh is slightly apart from your teeth and nothing is stuck inside your mouth. You may also shake just your lower jaw while producing a deep sound. This will have the effect of putting everything that is contained within your face in its proper place. When you finish the shake, put your head in the central balanced position, still on the floor, and relax.

The cheek shake should be performed not more than twice a week and preferably lying down.

Temporal and Frontalis Muscles

The temporal muscle has been described already (see page 94). It suffices here to add that the two temporal muscles are connected at the back of your skull. The frontalis muscle, which covers the central part of your forehead, travels upwards into your skull and may also be made to grow taller until it eventually reaches the crown area. For a perfect image of the direction towards which all forces should be pulling in these exercises, imagine a circus acrobat hung up by the ponytail performing all her wonderful tricks in this position. It is possible to guide minute muscle action by sheer will into a certain direction. Such action may not initially cause non-movable parts to move, but it will develop new muscle tissue. Repeated action directed towards a bodily part that cannot move with the intention of moving it will create new muscle tissue that will eventually be able to move previously static parts of a droopy face.

CHAPTER NINE

The Nose and Ears

The nose is not just a centre-stage feature in the face, it is a sensing organ which — with its little nostril hairs — helps us filter the air we breathe. Breathing in through the nose and out through the mouth is the best way to breathe. Your nostrils filter the air so that clean air goes into your body. When the air comes out it is dirty and you should expel it through your mouth.

Avoid bad smells and car fumes. Most importantly, if you do have to be in a smelly, stuffy environment, try to cover your nose and mouth with a clean handkerchief to filter out the bad air. When you do smell something unpleasant, immediately close your mouth so that at least the poisons won't enter your lungs through your throat. Allow your nostrils to filter the air but don't breathe deeply until the air is clear again. When you are walking in the city, always make sure you have a cotton scarf or handkerchief at hand to filter the foul air. To regain some of the original functions your nose was designed to have, indulge in smelling different types of herbs, flowers, oils and other scents that you find pleasant. Reduce the amount of salt you use in cooking and begin to appreciate the subtleties of smell.

Ear/Nose Connections

How to keep the nasal passage clean has already been dealt with in Chapter 4, Clean and Feed. In this chapter we consider how much a simple nose contraction can work to your advantage; we look at the internal ear/nose connections, and we discuss the shape of the nose, which people seem to worry so much about. The nose and ears are connected to the eyes and the mouth. When you cry, sneeze or massage the sinus area, you can feel these connections. The nose and ears are also connected to each other. To encounter this connection instantly, do the ear popping exercise (No.17) on page 75.

Nose Shape

The upper part of the nose is made of solid bone. The centre part is cartilage. The nostrils are made of very strong muscle. The muscle here is of almost of the same type as the anus or the mouth. Mobility in the nostrils has become almost dormant since humans have lost the need for finding food through the sense of smell, and the nostrils have become almost completely static. Nevertheless the origin of nostrils are ring muscles, and where there is muscle there is a way to change. Where there is no muscle, there is a way to create muscle. If you are really worried about your nose shape, don't rush to have a nose job done. Many of my friends who have suffered the pains of facial surgery came out of it much poorer and not necessarily better-looking. A large nose with a heavy fringe and a pair of spectacles stuck on top of it doesn't look very nice, but the same nose above a long neck, with hair combed back, is beautiful. Some of the most beautiful people have prominent noses. It is not so much the shape or size of a nose that matters, but how it is worn. You can even change the shape of your nose to a certain extent by a) making sure it is clear and unblocked, even in the uppermost part where swelling is often seen, and b) you can change your hairstyle to complement the shape of your nose. So before thinking about having a nose job done, read on . . .

I once found fortune in a small accident that occurred when my second son, then three years old, was sitting on my lap. He was wildly jumping about, as young boys do, when, with a sudden jerk of his head, he hit back and banged his skull full blast straight into the solid part of my nose. The impact was so great that I jumped up screaming, holding my nose, with tears pouring out of my eyes. Heavy bruising resulted from this accident and a few days later the pain had waned to a regular pulse. When I examined my nose after it had healed, I glided a finger downwards along its bridge and found, to my great surprise, that the small protrusion which had always been part of the shape of my nose was no longer there. It had disappeared! My nose has been straight ever since.

This incident was, in a way, a small version of what the plastic surgeon does to rebuild a nose, except that he does it a thousand times more violently under a general anaesthetic. The surgeon smashes a nose to bits with a hammer, keeping the air passages open, and then puts a beautifully shaped mould back onto the broken bone to make a new shape. Two weeks after the operation, the patient still looks like Quasimodo with a blue, green and purple swollen face, swallowing painkillers and recovering from major shock. Such a shock must cause irreparable damage to the system even if the act is performed under anaesthesia. Numbing the senses does not change the fact that there has been a major rupture in the body. One way or another, the body will have to cope with that.

(I) Exercise No. 55   Nose Contraction

Movement in the nose is very limited because, as mentioned earlier, we have no longer a use for the nose as a vital smelling organ. Nevertheless, it is possible to contract the flanks of the nose and, when performed correctly, the nose contraction constitutes one of the strongest multi-purpose toning exercises for the central part of the face. It will tighten your cheeks, work against a moustache line and at the same time, eliminate a frown.

Be very careful how you do it. Follow the instructions carefully and you won't go wrong.

A nose contraction can be performed either to good or to evil. If you wrinkle up your nose, you can see many little lines everywhere. Now perform the same action but make it smaller and control the creases; keep the skin smooth with the hands and you will find that this movement is quite easy to do and can be extremely powerful. Put the fingers on either side of the nose directly above the nostrils.

With a slight motion of the muscles above the upper lip, you will be able to make a movement with the flanks of your nose not unlike a sniffing dog, a nose contraction.

A similar sensation in the muscles involved can be felt when you perform a yawn with the mouth closed. My twin sister and I used to play this game when we were teenagers, travelling on long, boring train journeys. We would sit opposite each other in a full compartment when one of us would start. The movement is barely perceptible to an outsider, but if persistently sustained, contracting the flanks of your nose will cause the eyes to shed some tears. It is as if when the yawn cannot come out through the mouth, it will come out through the eyes instead.

The action is pressing upwards through the sinuses towards the eyes. It makes the nose more narrow at its base, directly above the nostrils, and it also tightens up the muscles holding the cheeks that are attached at that point to the nose. In addition, a snarl, or closed yawn, seems to excrete debris from the body, in the form of tears, which all helps to empty out puffed-up eyelids and overfilled eye bags you may have lying around on your face.

Hearing

Unless exercised, like all other bodily functions, the ears begin to weaken as age creeps up upon us. It is a good idea to check now how the ears work, before it is too late. If your ears are weak already, the following exercises will improve your hearing and stop the condition getting worse.

Ⓐ **Exercise No. 56** **Moving the Ears**

This co-ordination exercise is one of the most difficult ones to learn, but once it has become a natural part of facial vocabulary, it will help you lift the face instantly in any situation desired.

Some people can move their ears easily; others, the majority, to which I used to belong, find it impossible. The muscles to make the ears move are situated behind your ears, at the back of the skull. It seems that with extreme concentration, repetition, willpower and application, muscle activity can be created where previously none existed. You just have to try hard enough.

Start doing the exercise lying down flat on your back in the usual relaxed position. In this way you will not accumulate tension in your neck while practising.

1. Gently place three fingertips on your skull behind your ears.
2. Pull your fingers very slightly backwards towards each other and feel the ever so slight motion of the underlying musculature. As soon as you can feel the slightest movement, this will give you the proof and encouragement to pursue practising the exercise. This very tiny movement is the beginning of creating a strong band of flat muscle tissue which will span from ear to ear across the back of your head and serve as a natural "face hold" for the entire lower half of your face.
3. The feeling that accompanies movement of the ears — and I must admit that my own performance of it is still very mediocre — is similar to the feeling you have when you want to laugh, but a situation doesn't allow you to. You keep your mouth in its place with your lips closed, but something is pulling your ears back towards each other. Do this movement several times lying on your back and try to isolate it so as to not cause any contractions in the back of your neck.

Note: In the beginning when you are trying to move your ears you will find that all the muscles in your neck get involved, creating those wicked "guitar string" lines down the neck, so typical of uptight elderly women. If this occurs, you are on the wrong track for ear movement.

Tightening the muscles behind your ears will help you keep the jaw line smooth and the lower part of the chin, and side of the neck smooth and lifted at any time.

Hearing Threshold and Balance

How do you know when your hearing is good? When you find out it isn't, it's already too late. Test your hearing regularly. Do you have to make people repeat themselves when they speak to you because the way they pronounce words is unclear, or are you kidding yourself that your ears are perfectly all right? Weak hearing is such a common and impairing factor of ageing that we would all be well advised to take preventive measures before we begin to notice that people are avoiding talking to us.

Ⓑ **Exercise No. 57**

Finding the hearing threshold

You will need:

- a softly ticking watch
- some silence.

1. Sitting comfortably at the table, hold the watch at a distance far enough away from the right ear to lose its sound.
2. Bring the watch a little closer and notice at which point in space the sound becomes clear to you.
3. Move the watch further out again and mark in your vision the point at which the sound disappears.
4. Make the distance between the two points closer and closer until you are at a specific point in space between weak hearing and not hearing the sound at all. This is the hearing threshold of the right ear for that volume of sound.
5. Mentally measure the distance between your ear and that point (it may be between 6 and 12 inches (15-30 cm), depending on the sound level and your hearing power).

Performing the measuring exercise against a wall or blackboard allows you actually to draw the points.

Take the hearing threshold measurement for both ears.

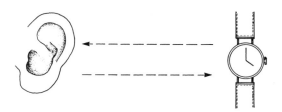

Fig 50: *Length of hearing threshold*

(I) Exercise No. 58   Tuning and Rebalancing the Ears

When you have found your hearing threshold, move your head slightly from side to side to find out which ear works best. If you can hear the sound better by turning your head to the right, but not so well when you turn to the left, that means that your left ear is weaker than the right one, and vice versa.

The disadvantage of unbalanced hearing is twofold:

a) It puts strain on your good ear and makes the weak ear even lazier. Unless this is treated with rebalancing exercises, your hearing will deteriorate further.

b) Imbalanced hearing will cause your head to be tilted to one side, this causes imbalance in the rest of your face. Imbalance in the carriage of your head affects your neck, shoulders, spine and can be perpetuated all the way down to the overall balance of the skeleton.

If you discover that one ear is weaker than the other you can begin training that ear to catch up with its twin.

This rebalancing exercise can be performed anywhere at any time. All you need is a degree of concentration.

1. Once you have established which ear is weaker, put the palm of your hand on your strong ear so as to create a kind of vacuum between your palm and the ear hole. You can hear the noise of your blood streaming through your head and hand. The harder you press, the louder the noise will become. Listen for a while, keeping the pressure strong enough to exclude as far as possible any real outside noise from that ear.
2. Now shift your concentration to your other ear, the one that is free but weak, and concentrate on the real outside noises that this ear absorbs. Feel the difference in sound between the ear that is covered and the free ear. Make a mental note of what the weak ear feels when it is active.

Experiment with using the weak ear more often than the strong ear. You could plug your strong ear for an entire afternoon or morning and you will find that your weak ear will become stronger. Once your ears are balanced, you may begin exercising both ears simultaneously to increase the power of your hearing further.

(I) Exercise No. 59   Stretching the Hearing Threshold

1. Find the threshold as in exercise No. 57.
2. Listen to the ticking watch at the existing threshold for a few moments.
3. Listen to the sound at a slightly more distant threshold until you are able to perceive the sound again.

If instruction number 3 is difficult, keep returning to the existing threshold, note the sound, remember it, lengthen the threshold and project the memorized sound into your ear. If you still can't hear it then repeat until you achieve results or, if there is still no improvement, go and have a good ear clean.

Speed of Hearing

As with all faculties in the body, speed of hearing is just as important as the level at which you can hear. The speed at which you are able to hear and select different kinds of noises will allow you in old age to enjoy birdsong and ignore aeroplanes. If you become one of the unfortunate people who have to go through life with an artificial hearing aid, you will soon find out that such machines amplify unwanted sounds, ignoring softness and beauty. Life can become very irritating indeed for these poor souls. So keep your ears fit while you can.

(A) Exercise No. 60

Speeding Up Hearing

You will need a metronome or other sound-making device of which the speed can be modified.

Take up any position, standing up, placed centrally and well balanced, sitting, or lying down, as you wish.

1. Switch on the sound source and listen to the repetitive sound waves. Absorb each sound as if it was new and you had never heard it before.
2. After about 30 seconds, speed up the sound and maintain the same concentration on each individual impulse.
3. Listen with one ear, with the other, then both. If you have a weak ear, listen with that ear again. Then listen with both again but being more conscious about the weak ear working as well. When you clearly hear the sound at this speed with both ears evenly, speed up the sound one mark faster. See how fast it goes before the individual sounds have all merged into a trill or a hum.
4. Finish the session with relaxation and breathing. Remember that the whole world is made up of different kinds of sound.

Look around you and notice how many objects emit sound. If you find any sound-producing machines in the house that have been left on for no reason, turn them off and enjoy the disappearance of an irritating sound. Like losing a louse on an itchy head, you get a sense of relief. Failing the total absence of sound in built-up areas, the best we can do is to pay attention to the small, pleasant noises so that later on in life, we will not have let them be overpowered by the unpleasant sounds of everyday life. Some people use earplugs when they go to bed. Personally, I can't bear them, as putting a stopper on my hearing faculty makes me feel very insecure and handicapped, when sleeping ought to be restful and regenerating.

(A) **Exercise No.61**   **Eargasm**

There is a small massage machine on the market designed to release neck tension. If you have such a machine, and it has a flat-on massage head, you may be one of the lucky people who can experience an eargasm.

1. Switch the machine on and place its head flat against your right ear, exactly where you placed your hand earlier to shut off the sound.
2. Now press the vibration deep down into your ear. Move the surface of the massager in small ironing motions until you find the position that allows the greatest penetration of soft vibrating sound to enter deep into your ear.
3. At the same time, make a deep growling sound with your own voice.

The resulting feeling, which I call an "eargasm", is a sudden connection felt between the vocal cords and the hearing canal, releasing a whole shower of accumulated tension in and under the jaw with the strength of a lavatory flush. The eargasm has been much enjoyed by many of my clients and is recommended when you suffer listlessness, have a clogged-up head and still want to get on with something. It will give you a real boost of power.

CHAPTER TEN

Mouth and Jaw

The mouth conveys your facial expression to other people. Look at your mouth in the mirror and notice its shape. Is the upper lip protruding or is the lower lip prominent? Does it have an overbite or an underbite? When your mouth is closed, is your lip line curled up, straight, or curling down? When you open your mouth to eat, speak, shout or laugh, is it symmetrical or do you lift up one side more than the other? In this chapter we examine the mouth and the jaw area with the aim of straightening up any irregularities; we will see how you can move your mouth and your jaw

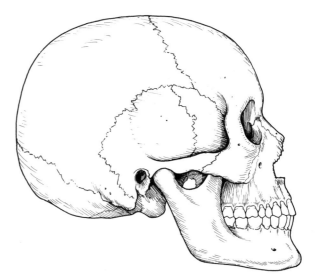

Fig 51: *The skull and the jaw*

economically but expressively, and we will discover how to get rid of unwanted bad habits. Firstly let us look at the alignment of the jaw in relation to the upper teeth.

The jawbone is the only bone in the head that can move independently of the skull. When you bite your food, the lower teeth make all the action while the upper teeth are static; they are rooted in the skull and have therefore no independent movement. Any movements made by your mouth are made by the muscles that control your jaw and the ring muscle around your lips.

When we chew food, the jaw moves in a combination of three basic moves, described below. Practise each of the moves independently to become aware of the full movement range of the jaw.

Jaw Movement

Like the lid on an inverted box, attached to the skull with hinges, the jaw can open and close itself. Without consciously lifting your lips, open your mouth as wide as possible and notice that the movement occurs in your jaw only. Your upper lip remains in place. Open and close your mouth several times to see that without moving the upper lip, the mouth can open itself down to quite a large opening. Practise opening and closing your jaw as wide as possible without making unnecessary lines.

Side to Side Jaw Movement

The jaw can move sideways to the right and left — rather as sheep or cows do when they are chewing food. With your teeth almost closed and your lips relaxed, move your jaw from side to side. You can feel that the action takes place somewhere beside your ears. Keeping this part of your face mobile and co-ordinated will help you execute many mouth corner lifting exercises, and help prevent premature deafness and loss of balance. It will also help to retain the mobility in the jaw, even if one or two teeth are missing. Do 50 repetitions of this movement without pulling down the corners of your mouth. When you are good at doing that and not too tired in the jaw, continue the sideways move, now with a slight smile. Lift the outer corners of your almost closed mouth and carry on chewing like a sheep for 50 more counts. Don't make any lines in the cheeks and around the mouth while practising. If necessary, use your hands at first to keep the skin smooth while you work. This will work as an excellent cheek toner as well as raising the corners of your mouth.

Protraction and Retraction of the Jaw (Forward and Backward)

The jaw can advance or retract, as can be so clearly seen in the overbite and the underbite.

To find out if you have an overbite or an underbite, do the following exercise.

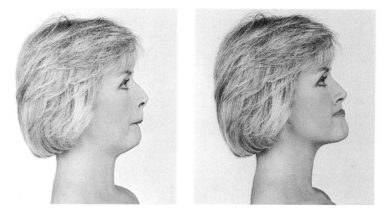

Fig 52: *Overbite and underbite*

Overbite and Underbite

Bite your molars together. Now notice the alignment of your front teeth. If the upper teeth overlap the lower teeth, you have an overbite. If the lower teeth overlap the upper teeth you have an underbite. Neither of these two positions are favourable assets to enhance beauty. The overbite makes you look stupid (don't ask me why) while the underbite makes a face look aggressive. Don't get discouraged if you have either of these two conditions, as it is relatively easy to straighten them out with the next exercise.

Ⓑ Exercise No. 62

Jaw Placement — The Cross Position

1. Place your two front upper teeth against the two central lower teeth so as to make a cross.

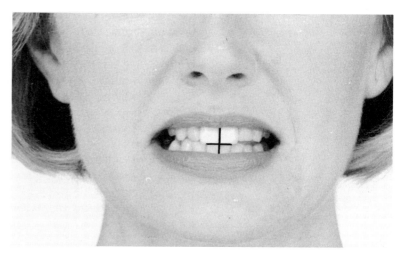

Fig 53: *Jaw alignment — the cross*

136

2. An index fingernail will help you hold the position if you feel it slipping away. Now don't let go of the cross even though it might feel to you as if you now have a crooked mouth. Check that everything looks straight; it only feels crooked because you are not used to holding the face in this way.
3. Hold the position with a minimum of muscular effort for a minute or two, and come back to this exercise if your mouth is very crooked, or if you have a strong over- or underbite.

Note: Be careful not to "bite" your teeth but just gently hold the four front teeth aligned in the cross position. Memorize the feeling of holding the jaw centrally, your front teeth barely touching, your mouth centred, closed and relaxed. It is only when you are able to hold the frame of your mouth in its correct alignment that you have a chance of placing the lips where they belong.

Teeth Trouble?

Regular visits to the dentist may be commonly recommended (by dentists) for good, healthy teeth. But have we not all suffered many a frightening and painful experience at the dentist? We are often advised to have teeth out to prevent further decay, and if the thought of dentures appals you, now is the time to discover what you can do to save your teeth from the dentist! In my personal opinion, dental treatment is often very harsh and completely unnecessary. In the case of teeth, as with other parts of the body, prevention is better than cure.

If your teeth are feeling painful or loose, take a tablet of pure calcium daily for one week and start chewing carrots, nuts and other raw, chewy or crunchy foods that you enjoy eating, like raw celery, courgettes, cauliflower, or red and green peppers. Within a few days of this regime, your teeth should be once again as firm as all the other teeth in your mouth. In addition you could try clacking your teeth 100 times a day for one week. Painful and decayed teeth must be treated, of course. But as I said, prevention is better than cure. Eating plenty of raw food, no sugar and, if possible, no meat, will keep your teeth strong and healthy for a long time to come. Apart from daily brushing, you should drink plenty of water after every meal (don't drink during the meal) and rinse your mouth out after eating. Use a natural hard brush to clean your teeth and always brush your tongue and gums with a slightly softer brush with soap and water. It doesn't taste very nice at first, but you soon get used to brushing your tongue and gums as part of everyday mouth care. Once in a while, about two or three times a week, it is a good idea to brush your teeth and gums with an electric toothbrush as this gives them a firming massage.

The worst thing for teeth is sugar and sticky sweet substances, as we all know. What is never mentioned, however, is that the fine fibres of meat is the next favourite foodstuff to collect between the teeth and in cavities. Meat is the most difficult to clean out when brushing. So if you were considering becoming a vegetarian and your teeth are in poor shape, this might give you another reason for stopping eating meat altogether.

If your teeth do begin to give you trouble I recommend that you examine your situation before going to an expert. You may be able to treat the problem yourself. If this is not the case, a thorough self-examination will help you explain the problem better to the dentist.

Checking for an Infection or Abscess

The word abscess is so very frightening and disgusting to many people that they immediately make an appointment to see the dentist, who, being an expert, is entrusted with the unwanted object.

Before you do this, next time your gums or teeth hurt, wash your hands in household antiseptic, go to a mirror by a sink with a bright light, open your mouth wide, and look inside.

Before pulling a cheek back to have a better look, rub lots of petroleum jelly on the area first. If there is an ulcer, a swelling, sometimes with a white or yellow pimple on top of it, then you don't need to go to the dentist at all.

Simply take a sharp object (sterilized or thoroughly disinfected) such as a very thin needle, which won't hurt, and very gently pierce a tiny little hole in the abscess. If the abscess is ripe, pus will come squirting out like a volcanic eruption.

With the cold water tap running, quickly press a cotton wool bud dipped in antiseptic on to the swelling and wash away the pus that comes out, until the swelling goes down and a little drop of blood appears.

Once the blood comes out, there is no more pus inside. Gargle and rinse your mouth out with a disinfectant mouth wash or just a few drops of antiseptic in a glass of water. Or if you have none of those at hand, just sprinkle some salt — a natural disinfectant — into a glass of luke warm water.

Note: Make sure you don't swallow any of the pus.

Helping yourself gives instant relief. Keep your mouth clean and you should be rid of your abscess. Had you gone to the dentist, you might well have had unnecessary X-rays and antibiotics, and probably had the tooth removed. Dentists are all very well in emergencies, but it is often perfectly possible to help yourself.

Lip Line Placement

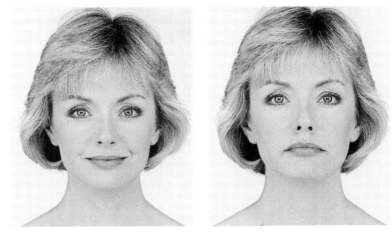

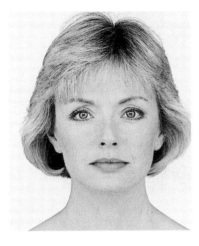

Fig 54: *lip line a) neutral, b) upward, c) downward*

To see how your lips are placed, you will need two mirrors at right angles to each other. As explained at the beginning of the book, the image you perceive of your face in a mirror is the reversed image of what another person sees or what a camera sees. Using two mirrors at right angles to each other gives you a picture that is equally accurate, yet less familiar to you. In the second mirror you will clearly see the asymmetry (unevenness) of the shapes in your face and this helps you work on the parts that most need rebalancing. The lip line placement exercise will show you that uneven lips can be made to look regular again by doing the exercises which follow.

Look at your mouth in the second mirror placed at a right angle to the first one. With the front teeth in their "cross" position, relax the lips and gently close them. Notice the shape of the line that separates the two lips and see which of the three shapes in Fig 54 it is closest to.

If the natural lip line is either like a) or b) in Fig 54, that is fine, but if you have a depressed lip line, then we have some work to do. In any event, even a neutral lip line or a permanently stuck grin can usefully do with the following mouth neutralizer.

Ⓑ Exercise No.63   Lip Line Placement

1. Align your jaw centrally, close your lips and mark a straight line on the mirror with a felt tip or a piece of tape. The line should be absolutely horizontal.
2. Now draw another line vertically across this line to form a long cross and align the centre of your lips, the tip of your nose, the point centrally situated between the eyebrows and the top of your head with the vertical line.

3. Match your lip line to the straight horizontal line and hold it without tension for 10 counts.
4. Begin widening your closed mouth gradually sideways, but keep the line horizontal.

   One mouth corner may begin to shake a little as its muscles are not used to being held in this position. The challenge, then, is to retain the position without moving a muscle. The position you are holding now is the neutral or straight lip line position. If you can hold it for more than 20 counts, try.
5. When you feel the hold tensing up too much or slipping away, release your muscles, a few at a time, to come to a halt and relax your mouth.

Repeat the alignment and as soon as you've got it, walk away from the mirror, retaining the shape of your mouth. Go and do something casual, like washing your hands, or tidying up something, while trying to retain the neutral lip alignment. Then come back to the mirror to see if the neutral position is still there. You will probably find that it has sagged again so begin once more until soon, this neutral position will be easy to hold. Hold your mouth in the neutral position for an increasing number of counts every time you practise this exercise. If it won't stay there by itself, you may use your hands to help you but eventually you should be able to hold your mouth in its neutral position with its own muscles, without twitching or shaking.

You may keep the two lines on the mirror for daily use in rebalancing the position of your mouth and as a general check for facial alignment.

When you are able to achieve a straight lip line, you may progress to embellishing its shape. A mouth can go either of two ways from its horizontal, neutral position. It can turn into a smile, or it can turn into a villain's mouth, with the corners drooping down. Certain mouths are shaped with a slight turn up of the corners naturally. Babies and young children's mouths tend to be like that. Look around and notice among all the faces you see in any one day: see which mouths are neutral, turned up or turned down and judge for yourself which you find more attractive. Some people seem to manage a smile even when they are upset or angry, especially on TV sit-coms and other popular forms of entertainment, but a permanently stuck grin can be most irritating. The subtlety of an ever-so-small degree of turn up in the outer corner of your lips is very fine indeed and will only look natural if it is a result of permanent muscle tone, rather than muscle action. But since muscle action creates muscle tone, now you can go ahead and design yourself some pretty lips.

Ⓑ Exercise No. 64   Curling Up the Mouth

Lie down on your back and relax your cheeks, neck, shoulders and your whole face. Again, align your teeth centrally in the cross position, close your lips and relax. Feel the sides of your mouth pulling down towards your ears.

1. Enhance this gravitational pull with your own muscular action by pushing your jaw forward completely so that your lower lip wraps over your top lip, and slowly form a smile.
2. Take a deep breath and hold the slightly pulled-up mouth corners for eight counts.
3. Now direct your energy towards the very extremities of the mouth corners and pull them up higher and tighter.

   Hold the position for eight counts, release step by step for eight counts and relax.

Watch your face in a hand mirror while doing this to make sure no lines are created anywhere on the face while you are working.

Ⓘ Exercise No.65   Mouth Corner Toner

1. Still lying on your back, make a small "O" shape with your mouth and smile.
2. Pull up the mouth corners up 75 times or more until the muscles outside the mouth corners become tired and limp.
3. Finish the sequence by speeding up the contractions and making them smaller and smaller, until your mouth corners are almost shaking. Breathe deeply and ever so slowly release the muscles that have been working so hard. You will find that your mouth will want to stay in this position for ever, but instead, give the area a shake and a gentle massage to allow all the tension to flow away.

Erasing Lines on the Upper Lip

The following four exercises are designed to erase the nasty little lines on the upper lip. If you smoke, often drink from straws, kiss small kisses, and whistle a lot, you are more likely to have these lines than if you don't do those things. Apply petroleum jelly to your lips and massage them soft and warm before you begin.

Ⓑ Exercise No.66   Erasing Lines on the Upper Lip (1)

1. Grip the upper lip with the thumb and forefinger of each hand and knead the upper lip while slightly pulling it outwards to get blood flowing through all its parts.
2. Massage the inside of the top lip as much as the outside until it becomes warm and supple.
3. When you rest from this massage and manipulation, place the lips again in their neutral position, aligning the teeth centrally and practise lifting the mouth corners.

Ⓑ Exercise No.67   Erasing lines on the upper lip (2)

Whether you can actually whistle or not is immaterial for this exercise. Look in the mirror and whistle, or pretend to whistle if you can't. Notice the shape that your mouth is in. If you are making wrinkles in the upper lip, change its position, with your fingers if necessary, and whistle some more without making lines in the upper lip. I used to enjoy whistling long melodies and was quite good at it until I tried this exercise which is a combination of everything we have done so far for the mouth.

1. Make a small oval-shaped mouth with a slight upward lift of the mouth corners, and whistle a tune without wrinkling the upper lip. Good luck!
2. If it won't work first time, use the hands in this most intricate piece of facial contortion. If you are able to perform this combination of movements without making any grimaces or lines on the face and without the help of the hands, you can call yourself a black belt in facial exercise. Don't forget to relax the forehead and not to frown while you are practising.

Ⓘ Exercise No.68   Erasing Lines on the Upper Lip (3)

Another factor which causes wrinkles on the top lip to appear is the way we speak. Stand in front of the mirror and produce the letter "O", now the letter "U". Say the word "Howard" and observe the contraction that the upper lip is making. If you see any small lines appearing at all, practise saying the sounds without making the lines. The tiny muscle units that form the large ring muscle of the mouth will learn to work together more evenly without creasing. A good sequence to practise saying would be:

Repeat the sounds "O", "U" and "how" 15 times each, checking the shape of the upper lip. Hands may be used if the lip is not willing to stay smooth, but as usual, diminish hand aid as soon as possible.

Now formulate all the vowels and consonants keeping a close watch on your mouth, making sure it does not pull off-centre or wrinkle at any time. In this way you will learn to formulate words without creating unnecessary wrinkles.

Ⓐ Exercise No.69   Erasing Lines on the Upper Lip (4)

The point in the cleft midway between the bottom of the nose and the centre of the top lip is called in acupressure Ren-Zhong; it is the emergency point for fainting, dizziness and nausea. It is also, not surprisingly, the point little children always put their finger on when they are feeling lost or insecure.

Put the soft part of your index finger on the cleft. Open your jaw wide, keeping your lips over your teeth. Now press down hard on the cleft while smiling. Contract your top lip against the resistance of your finger so that your mouth forms a heart shape. Be careful not to crease the moustache line while doing this exercise. Use your other hand if necessary.

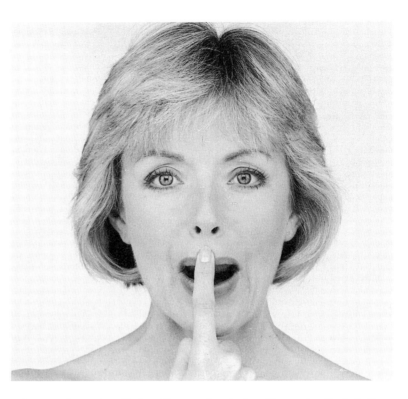

Fig 55: Upper lip line eraser

Repeat the action 30 slow times or less but until your top lip feels limp from working and stretching its medial part.

Laughing and Smiling

In movement dynamics the action of laughing could be compared to that of jumping. Your cheeks are thrown in the air with rapid thrusting movements in the back of your throat, propelled by the voice. Air is expelled from your lungs which makes your vocal cords vibrate, thus producing sound. Laughing may be done in many different ways and although it seems a paradox to have to lay down rules about a function as spontaneous as laughing, doing so will save your face from major damage. The action of laughing is the largest and fastest of all facial movements and therefore needs particular attention if we want to restore a balanced face. Laughing is perhaps, after sexual orgasm, the nicest feeling a body can experience. Laughing is contagious. Laughing is fun, but if you are caught in a laughing attack which is out of control you may end up creating too many lines on your face — and the lines might become permanent one day if you carry on like that. We have already seen on the

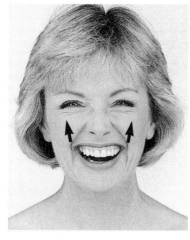

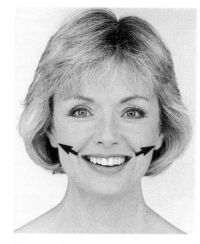

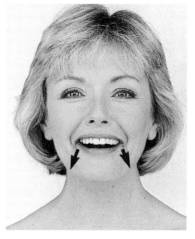

a) towards the temples/eyes (incorrect)

b) towards the earlobes (correct)

c) towards the shoulders (incorrect)

Fig 56: *Laughing*

face wrinkle map that wrinkles can be either positive or negative. Now we should study how we laugh and adjust the movement patterns to create an expression of laughter which does not produce a distorted face.

The trick in laughing is to direct the contractions outwards towards your ears and the corners of your jawbone rather than either towards your temples or your eyes, or even worse, pulling the laughing muscles down towards your shoulders which creates "guitar strings" down your neck and drooping mouth corners. Adopt the correct laughing position as illustrated in Fig 56 and hold it for two minutes. You may continue doing anything else you wish to do during that time!

Ⓘ Exercise No.70 Laughing

Notice the difference in the three laughs in Fig 56 and practise the one in the middle, (b). While you practise this position make sure your eyes remain wide open and your forehead relaxed. Memorize the muscle units at work in this practice position. Make a mental note of the difference between how you laugh habitually and this position. In time, if you keep on practising various degrees of smiles, with or without any accompanying laughing noises, even the most spontaneous outbursts will adopt the correct movement patterns.

Ⓐ Exercise No.71 Laugh Again

Catch yourself laughing spontaneously and notice all the lines above your cheeks and the crow's feet in the corner of your eyes. If you are a nose wrinkler, there are also lines between your eyebrows and even, perhaps, on the forehead. The object of this exercise is to laugh out loud with the minimum amount of lines created.

Begin to practise the laugh from the neutral mouth position described earlier. Make sure your face is well creamed or oiled so that your skin is soft before you start.

1. From the neutral position, while relaxing the rest of your face, pull the corners of your mouth out towards your ears. Make sure you do not create lines while doing so. Check that your teeth are aligned properly in the "cross" position in the centre.
2. Continue pulling your mouth corners outwards towards your earlobes. One or both sides of the mouth may be slightly shaky. If this happens, maintain the position at which the shake begins and stay there for 16 counts. Now pull the corners out further and begin to produce a laughing sound. Don't release the laugh abruptly, but come back to normal slowly and gradually, and try to retain some of the joyful expression of laughter in your eyes and on your face for good.

The Moustache Line

The moustache line is the diagonal wrinkle going from the top of each nostril down towards the mouth corners. They are always created when laughing or shouting. These lines are more prominent in skinny people, and give people an air of being worn out and permanently angry. There are some good techniques to eliminate the moustache line, as you will see in the following exercises.If the muscles underneath are well toned, the lines will only appear in movement, and they won't create deep wrinkles which eventually lead to a complete cheek fold.

Ⓑ Exercise No.72

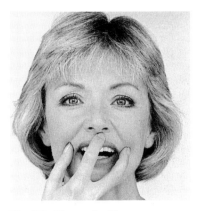

Fig 57: *Moustache line eraser*

Moustache Line Eraser

Place the index finger on the cleft, the thumb and third finger on either mouth corner as illustrated.

1. Open your mouth a little and smile. Now keep repeating the smiling contraction against the resistance of your fingers placed on the upper lip. You will see that the line that normally appears when you laugh has now turned into a mere gentle dimple.
2. Repeat the contraction 50 times and feel the whole upper lip area toning up. Massage the lip after you finish and keep your face relaxed but remember the feel of the muscles you have just been using.

This exercise is particularly useful for diminishing the moustache line, as the contraction works right into the crease of the line itself, thereby toning tiny muscles that have been deprived of action for a long time. Toning these will fill up the deep groove of the moustache line.

Drinking Movements

Drinking is more than quenching thirst. Alcohol is the most accepted form of drug taking and therefore holding a drink, even if it does not contain alcohol, has turned into a social mode of expression. If the movement patterns in drinking are poor it will not only create an ugly face in future years, but it will also diminish your beauty now. To check that you drink gracefully, go and stand by the two mirrors at right angles to each other so that you are able to see your face in profile. Now observe how you drink a glass of water. Do you pucker your top lip forward? Are your teeth out of alignment? Is your jaw retracted? Drink again, but this time keep the teeth aligned in the "open cross" position and don't make a puckered top lip and don't create lines on it. Keep your top lip in line with your bottom lip. Concentrate both on the image in the mirror and on the feeling in your muscles while you are correcting the action. You may find that the bottom lip is unnecessarily curled while you drink, which will create a line above the chin. Turn the other way round and look at the picture from the other side. Check again that you are not retracting the jaw, making a double chin or any other nasty movements that you can avoid making while drinking.

Finally, if you are not sure what to do with the mouth, keep smiling an invisible internal smile, through thick and thin, and I promise you, fortune will not fail to come your way.

CHAPTER ELEVEN

Shoulders, Neck and Chin

Neck and Shoulder Tension

Most people tend to hold considerable tension in the top part of the back of the neck, and in the shoulder region. Restriction of movement in the neck, as explained earlier, causes muscles to be permanently contracted without ever stretching to their naturally designed length. Tension, headaches, migraine and irritability are the well-known ailments which are caused at least in part by tension in the neck and shoulders. Any tension area can be likened to a blocked drain between the head and the spine which prevents easy transport of electricity, chemicals and nutrients between the brain and the rest of the body.

Men who wear stiff shirts and ties, the accepted attire for leading male figureheads, are particularly prone to tension. A collar and tie restricts free movement of the head. Instead of turning his head in order to look round, a shirt-and-tie-wearer will often turn his torso and shoulders because his neck can hardly move. Generals, presidents, popes and princes, politicians, professors, lawyers, doctors and businessmen all wear this restricting dress. Even Third World countries and Japan have adopted it. And if the head cannot turn, then how is it possible to appreciate a full circular horizon from a strong and balanced central viewpoint?

An average person's vocabulary of regular daily movements entails mostly moving the hands, the face and the head, a little walking and much

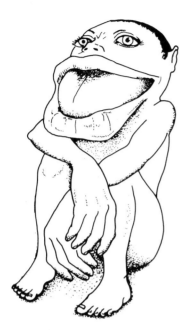

Fig 58: *The anamorphic man*

sitting. The anamorphic man illustrates this perfectly. The anamorphic man was a sculpture of the human body with its bodily parts blown up or reduced in size to the degree with which they are used. The resulting sculpture looked like Fig 58.

The head on the drawing is the largest part, after the hands and the mouth. The trunk and limbs are virtually nonexistent because they are rarely used. The feet are also quite small. We use our hands and arms all day long, holding things — pencils, knives and forks — carrying things — briefcases and shopping and umbrellas, hats and gloves and scarves and parcels, and manoeuvring things — travel tickets, bank cards, calculators and microcomputers. Manipulating all day, we are not only using the muscles in our fingers and hands: the muscles along our arms, shoulders and the upper back are always involved. When lifting a suitcase, we even use our abdominal muscles, the muscles of our ribcage, waist, hips and thighs. After the shoulders and neck, the second most common tension spot is the groin. People carry a lot of tension on the inside of the hip. Women especially carry deep tension in the pelvic basin. This could be attributed to the way women have always been brought up to keep the legs held tightly together and also to sitting habits.

A muscle that is never allowed to feel its length can never reach out for energy from other parts of the body. If a muscle is active, as they are in most day-to-day movement, but never stretched out to its full potential movement range, it turns into what an osteopath once called "old rope" muscles. Like a prisoner, the muscle is stiff, lacks blood, is weak. To revitalize such a piece of old rope, all you need to do is to move the bone upon which the muscle rests into a position that will allow the muscle to reach its full length. Rest and breathe in that position for a while and enjoy the energy flowing back into the muscle all by itself. Once a muscle has been lengthened in a good stretch, it is capable of being toned. If the muscle is never stretched, however, it will never be fully alive; even if it is toned, it will stay short and deprived of blood.

Upside Down Test

If you suspend a person upside down by the ankles and let them hang freely in space, it becomes apparent that very often one arm seems shorter than the other. The bone structure is not shorter, but the way in which the muscles are tensed, from repeated action in that particular arm, makes the arm so rigid that it remains in a permanent shortened state. A right-handed person, for example, usually has a shorter right arm. It will also emerge that the same side of the body carries the most neck and shoulder tension. If you are right-handed you should try to use the left hand more often (and vice versa for left-handed people), in order to rebalance this division between right and left in all the muscles in the body.

The shoulders and the neck are the pedestal for the head. It is therefore absolutely crucial that the upper back and neck are held in an erect position to give the most efficient form of support for the head. The external appearance of a neck can only be improved if there is a neck there to work on. Many people who come to the dance studio appear to have no neck, because they bury them between their chins and shoulders. I don't blame them in the constant drizzle and cold wind of a dark London winter, but postures like this can soon become permanent features. The first way to deal with the neck is to avoid bad movement, and the next stage is to strengthen the muscles in the neck so that they may be able to hold the head up high without having to resort to bad movement. To become fully aware of your neck, do Exercise 74, the Neck Lengthener.

How To Wear Clothes

Whenever possible, leave your neck free from tight collars, scarves, and heavy necklaces. Ageing women tend to hide their necks as this area is often the first place to wrinkle, even before the eyes, mouth or forehead. However, as the head is moving all day long and the neck turning and twisting constantly, cumbersome clothing can hinder movement. The friction of material, especially synthetic material, has many adverse

a) incorrect   b) correct

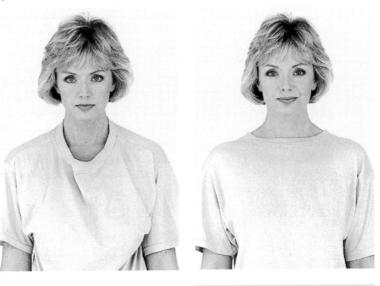

Fig 59: *How to wear clothes*

effects: it constantly wipes the skin dry, hinders free access of air, becomes uncomfortable and prevents free movement, thereby further stiffening the muscles of the neck. Temperature and pollution permitting, never cover your neck above the clavicles, upper back and trapezius.

Compare the two illustrations in Fig 59. The first one will be pulling down towards the front, stopping any possibility of moving the back of the neck where it should be placed. Heavy coats with large, weighty collars contribute further towards an already imbalanced posture. Looking at the body from above, the collar should be centred around the line of gravity.

Shoulder Bags

Wearing a shoulder bag forces the muscles on one shoulder to be perpetually contracted, thereby pulling one shoulder up. It is not possible to carry a shoulder bag on a relaxed shoulder: it would fall off. Permanently lifting a shoulder causes unnecessary tension in the neck and shoulder on the side the bag is worn. If you must have a shoulder bag, wear it across the opposite shoulder so that, at least, its weight is more centrally distributed. As this can get in the way of a voluptuous bust and also looks rather like a boy scout you may, in the end, decide to just get rid of the shoulder bag altogether. As you begin to need less make-up, you may be able to do away with a handbag full of junk. Wearing handbags full of junk is only a sign of insecurity anyway. Do you really need one? A little money, car keys and a few credit cards surely can easily fit into a pocket instead, leaving your arms free when walking in the streets. There is no reason why we should always have to clutch on to something, simply out of habit.

Aside from the fact that neck movement may be hindered through clothing, particular attention should be paid to the lower cervical vertebrae. To understand which part of the neck we are dealing with here, imagine that you are a kitten that is being picked up by its mother, and allow the back of your neck to come out. Only then will you ever be able to move the neck freely.

When you look up, for example, or when you bend your head backwards, what exactly happens in the vertebrae of your neck?

Ⓑ **Exercise No.73**   **Looking Up**

Stand up straight and bend your head back to look up to the sky. Does the back of your head rest in the "lap" of your shoulders? Compare the two illustrations in Fig 60 and see which you like best.

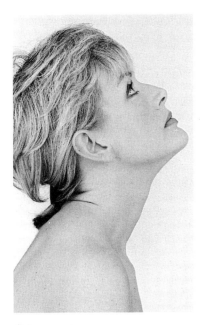

a) incorrect

Fig 60: *Looking up/bending the head back*

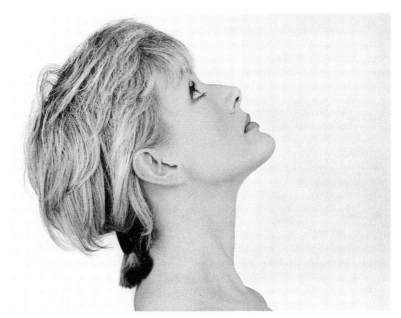

b) correct

Look up high eight times without creating any lines in the back of your neck. You may not be going very far at first, but at least you will keep your neck free and strengthen its muscles.

Whenever during the course of the day you look up or bend your head back to drink, make sure you don't create a broken neck line in the process. Illustration (a) shows that the subject's neck muscles are too weak to hold the head in an upward position, so the shoulders have been raised to take the weight of the head. That in itself tenses up the shoulders, but what happens to the neck itself in this incorrect position is that it gets curved in and jammed. This situation creates many knots and tension spots in the back of the neck. It is very important when you exercise the neck to keep it in one piece and not to create a broken neck line.

① Exercise No.74   Neck Lengthener

Whether you have a short neck or a long one, gravity is pushing the weight of your head down all day, so it is a good idea to lengthen the neck daily when you wake up and before you go to sleep, or at any other time when your neck feels stiff. And what better way to lengthen your neck than to hang your head upside down, like a dead turkey.

Stand with your back close to a full-length mirror, your feet slightly apart in the usual standing position with your arms relaxed.

1. Slowly bend your head down, then your neck, shoulders, ribcage, waist and finally your pelvis, until your hands loosely touch the floor and

your head is freely hanging in space. Through your legs, you can now see your head upside down in the mirror. Keep your legs straight if you can. If not, bend your knees a little.

2. Very gently shake your head as if to say "no" and feel your neck getting longer from the downward-pulling weight.

   Note: If you feel uncomfortable with the blood and oxygen rising to your head, *slowly* come up, working yourself up from your pelvis, going through your waist, ribcage, shoulders, neck and head in that order. You will only get dizzy if you perform the movement too quickly. Getting a little dizzy is not harmful: it helps you find a better sense of balance. Take a deep breath as you come up and exhale when you get to the top.

3. Now that you are up again, imagine that someone is pulling your crown upwards, straight up towards the ceiling.

4. Drop your shoulders and leave your arms limp and relaxed by the side of your body.

In this erect position, with a long neck, feel the back of your neck pulling upwards and backwards. your chin should be held down, the focus slightly up. In the upright position, again perform the "no" movement gently from side to side so that you are not able to see any part of your body except the top of your shoulders at the sides of your downward vision. Look down with your eyes but don't bend your neck down. Keep your head in the correct position, centrally placed above your spine. Slowly repeat from the beginning a couple of times until you feel quite happy with hanging upside down and no longer feel any discomfort or dizziness. It is a wonderful restorative to do the neck lengthener whenever your neck feels stiff or when you are tired.

Ⓑ Exercise No.75 Toning the Neck

The skin on the front part of your neck is very thin: at its worst it can look like a turkey pouch, at its best like the skin on the inside of a healthy young forearm, where the skin is of the same thickness and texture. To keep the skin of your neck beautiful and supple you will have to deal with it in several ways. Firstly, as you improve the carriage of your head and the way you move your neck and your head generally, you will learn to avoid making movements that create ugly lines. For example, retracting your chin too far back, as in an underbite, creates lines under the chin and in the hollow part under the jawbone at the top side of the neck.

1. Perform each position (see p.87) while massaging oil, cream or nutrient into the neck, chin and shoulder area. Don't forget your back.

2. Every time you clean your face, finish off by splashing or tapping the front of your neck and the lower part of your chin, again, moving through the basic neck positions.

The combination of movement, massage and toning is what creates such fast rejuvenating results in the condition of your neck. It is therefore vital to move your neck through all of its correct positions while you work on your skin.

Double Chin

A double chin can do so much damage to the beauty of a face, as it ruins the harmony of the natural shape of the skeleton. A double chin can be caused by lack of movement, being overweight or incorrect carriage of the head. Whatever the cause may be, it can be corrected with chin ups and the other exercises that follow.

Ⓑ Exercise No.76   Chin Ups on the Floor

The chin up exercise reduces a double chin in the same way as a sit up can reduce and tone up the stomach. So if you have a double chin and want to get rid of it, this is how to start.

Lie down on your back on the floor in the usual relaxed position, knees pulled up, hands down by the side.

1. Lift your head (and *only* your head) as far up as it will go.
2. Gently put it down again.
   You should be breathing out through your mouth as your head comes up and breathing in through your nose as you put it down.
   This exercise will be strenuous on your neck so you should do it slowly, and rest your neck fully on the floor after every chin up.
3. Repeat five times only for the first time, then as many as you can manage before going purple in the face and exploding!

Ⓘ Exercise No.77   Chin Ups in Space

Chin ups in space is a more advanced version of the chin up exercise and should only be done when the chin ups on the floor have been well mastered.

1. Lie down on your back at the top of a clean and well-carpeted staircase, with your neck and head hanging freely in space as in Fig 61.
   Make sure that your back is not hollow. If it is, place a small cushion just under your tail bone and pull up your knees; this will straighten your pelvis.
2. Now feel the heavy weight of your head pulling down until you can rest it either in the cup of your clasped hands, or on the next step down on the stairs. Keep your neck in one piece, bending back from your upper back.

Fig 61: *Chin ups in space*

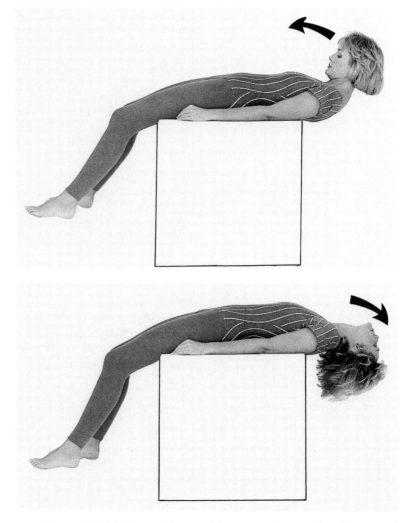

If you find this impossible to achieve or very uncomfortable, go and get some cushions and prop yourself up until you can comfortably lie down, making sure that you are doing it correctly, without breaking the neck line.

3. Now from this backward position, lift your head slowly and put it down again. You suddenly become aware that your head is exceptionally heavy.

4. Do five slow chin ups if you can. Rest and breathe, rub the back of your neck and repeat the sequence, this time with seven chin ups. Don't do more than seven the first time. When you repeat the exercise tomorrow you may increase the number of chin ups to 10 or 15 but always make sure you finish with a full neck relaxation.

Chin ups are one of the heaviest exercises to do at first because we are not used to carrying the full weight of our head in or below the horizontal plane. If you can't manage chin ups in space, go back to the chin up exercise on the floor until your neck muscles have gained some strength. Chin ups illustrate perfectly how much weight the muscles of your upper back, shoulders and neck are having to carry all day long when the head is held in an unbalanced position and at an angle in front of the body.

To reduce tension in your upper back and neck, always hold your head high and balanced when sitting or standing, and as soon as you feel that your neck is getting tired, lay your head down to rest. Who said *homo sapiens* had to live upright all the time?

Neck Articulation

The lateral range of movement in the neck can be measured with your vision. In order to increase further your balance and centring, stand up with your feet slightly apart and do the following exercise to loosen up a stiff neck and to measure and expand your horizon.

1. Turn the head to its extreme "no" position towards the right and note what is the furthest object you can see in the sideways periphery of your vision behind you on the right side. If your horizon is a flat clock the centre of which is your head, how far clockwise can you see: four, five, or six o'clock — right behind you? Remember not to cheat and to move your neck only, not your shoulders.
2. Now turn to the other side and note how far you can see. Can you recognize objects behind you that you saw on the right?
3. Still leading with your head, loosely swing your body from side to side. looking back as far as you can. Leave your arms relaxed. They will flow with the movement. Now you are not only stretching the sideways periphery of your vision, you are also twisting your torso, which is very good for the spine, as long as you maintain a perfectly upright position. Keep your feet, ankles and knees firmly facing the front. The movement should start at the waist and not lower, or you might dislocate your knee joints and that won't help your face at all.
4. Perform 8 or 16 such twists, slowing down as you reach the end, your arms still dangling freely. Take a deep breath, find your bearings, and rotate your head twice slowly, to one side, and then the other. Keep your eyes closed and your neck very relaxed as you go round.

(A) **Exercise No.78**   **The Bench Treatment**

The bench treatment is a further progression of the chin up exercise and works not only for the neck and chin, but also loosens a stiff upper back,

Fig 62: *The bench treatment*

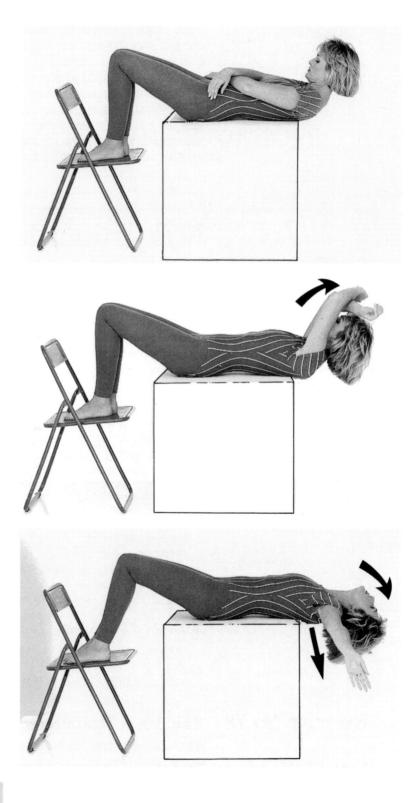

aching shoulder joints and strengthens weak stomach muscles. When you do this exercise for the first time, make sure there is someone nearby to help you in case you can't do it properly. You will need a bench or a single bed and a full-length mirror. If you use a bed, place it parallel to the mirror and lie across it on your back.

Place a bench at right angles to the full-length mirror and lie on it with your head towards the mirror. Keep your feet on or near the ground. If the back of your waist curls up too much, place a small hard cushion under your tail bone. Your upper back, from just above the shoulder blades, should be hanging freely in space. Only go as far as you can comfortably hold and allow your head to hang down backwards. Raise your arms behind you, so that they are hanging by your ears. Now gently shake your head from side to side.

1. Breathe in, and on the out breath, slowly lift your chin towards your breastbone. At the same time bring your hands towards your belly, crossing them over on their upwards path.
2. Breathing in slowly, go back down on to the bench. Lift your crossed hands high up above your head and spread them out sideways as you go down, back to the starting position.
3. Relax backwards with your head hanging down in space. Make sure that you bend from the upper back and not from the base of the neck. You may repeat this slowly 15 to 20 times until the neck becomes stronger. When you get tired, just pause where you are, hanging, relaxing your neck, face and scalp in the back and downward position.

When you become more comfortable with this exercise, you will be able to perform many of the facial exercises in this position, with your face hanging upside down, looking into the mirror and having a jolly good back stretch at the same time. The advantage of doing the exercises upside down is that in this position you use the antagonist muscles (antagonist = a muscle that opposes the action of another) to those you use normally to attain a position, attacking gravity from both ends. This is how, now that you have progressed further into the facial and postural exercises, you are now able to combine exercises to save you time and increase their potency. In this way you are not only achieving faster results, but the work also becomes easier all the time.

(A) Exercise No. 79 Advanced Chin Ups

Advanced chin ups should not be performed by people who are unable to do at least 15 slow sit ups on the floor. A lesser state of fitness in the stomach muscles would not allow them to get out of the position and they may get stuck there, fall down, break a leg and sue me for damages. So don't do it, unless you are capable of getting out of it.

Lying on the bench or across the bed as in the previous exercise, put your hands under the back of your head with the fingers interlocked. Pull your head out and backwards in space to lengthen your neck. The effort

Fig 63: *Horizontal head, neck and spine alignment*

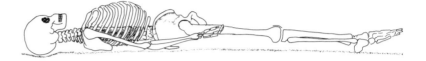

should come from the arms only. Don't point your chin upwards — this creates tension in the back of the neck.

1. With your head held in a perfect horizontal position in space, turn it to the side (the "no" movement) and check in the mirror the straight alignment of your head and neck. If correct, your neck should be in line with the bench and the "cup" of the back of your skull just below that line as illustrated.
2. Now turn your head back to the front and remove your hands while maintaining this exact position.
    Note: If it is too heavy, don't let go with your hands completely until your neck gets strong enough. Your head feels so heavy that you will only be able to hold it for a second or two at first.
    As you get stronger, practise slow "no" movements in horizontal space once a fortnight. Always do as many as you can (between 5 and 10) plus a few more that you couldn't do before.
3. To end the sequence, drop the entire upper back, neck and head down towards the floor, and relax. Let your arms hang down freely. Breathe deeply for about 10 slow breaths. Slowly come out of the position into a sit up. Support your head again with your clasped hands and roll up from that point, through your neck, shoulders, ribcage, waist and pelvis in that order until you are again sitting in an upright position on the bench.

Shoulders and Arms

The importance of shoulder placement as a base for a good face cannot be emphasized enough. You may have the most beautiful pair of eyes, but if your head rests on a stoop or a hunch, if your shoulders are hanging in front of you or pulled tightly backwards, you are carrying so much tension that you will not come across as truly beautiful. Several shoulder exercises are given here to help you keep your shoulders well placed, loose and strong.

The correct place for your shoulders is at the side of your body: not in front and not behind. To test your shoulder alignment, lie down on the floor with your knees pulled up and your head resting flat. Are your shoulders resting on the floor, or are they lifted off the floor? Keep your arms straight and your hands resting by your sides, and spread your fingers, tracing a semi-circular path along the floor up towards your head. On this path of movement, take a slow in breath. Stop the movement anywhere on its path and breathe out. Relax your shoulder muscles and feel your shoulders sinking down deeper towards the floor on each out breath. You mustn't push or force your shoulders down as this will create tension; let gravity do all the work for you. If the TV was built into the ceiling, you could lie there, slowly moving and stopping at various intermediate stages of this circular path while watching your favourite programme. It would help realignment of your shoulders to adopt some of these positions when going to sleep. But as most beds are jammed against a wall, usually with a headboard, the pleasure of fully stretching our arms above our head in sleep has also been taken away from us by the civilization of furniture. I sleep on a carpet on the floor myself and cannot bear sleeping in a bed. When you have explored the full range of your shoulder joints on the floor, stand up again. To loosen them up fully, do the following shoulder swings.

Shoulder Articulation

Shoulder placement has already been dealt with in Chapter 1, Self-image. Here, we are dealing with articulation, or how to move your shoulders to keep them supple enough to keep them in their correct place, without causing undue tension. Most of the tension that causes stiff necks, headaches, digestive and respiratory problems lies in the shoulder region. As we have seen earlier, connections between the face, neck and shoulders go as far down as the back, and through the arms into the hands and fingers. It is therefore important to relax your hands when they are not needed as doing so will release tension in your shoulders and neck. The following series of exercises are all geared to loosen and strengthen the shoulder joints, arms, hands and fingers.

Ⓑ Exercise No.80

Shoulder Stretch

1. Lie on one side with your knees pulled up as in Fig 64. Your arms should rest on the floor at shoulder height, palms down on the floor. Relax, but try to keep both shoulders on the floor.
2. Breathe deeply and slowly for 30 to 60 counts. There might be a slight pull on the front part of your left shoulder. Allow this lengthening to happen a little further with each out breath.
3. Roll over to the other side, by bringing your knees high up above your chest without moving your hands and shoulders.
4. Repeat the shoulder stretch on the left. Whereas a toning exercise needs repeating many times to strengthen a muscle, a stretching exercise only has to be done once or twice, until the extremity of a

Fig 64: *Shoulder stretch*

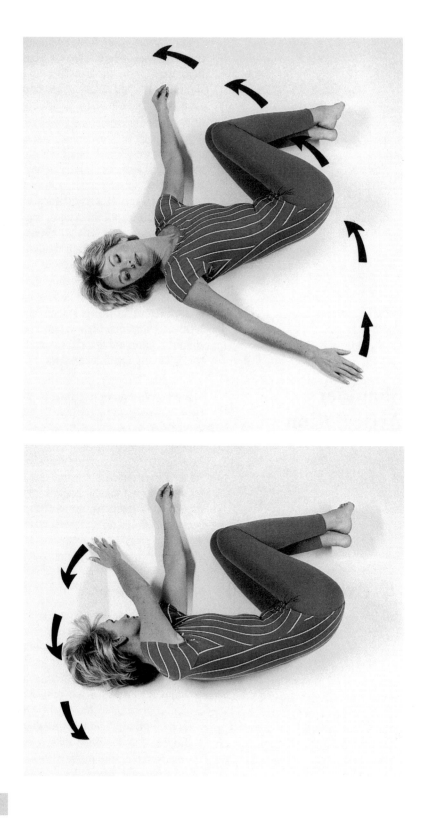

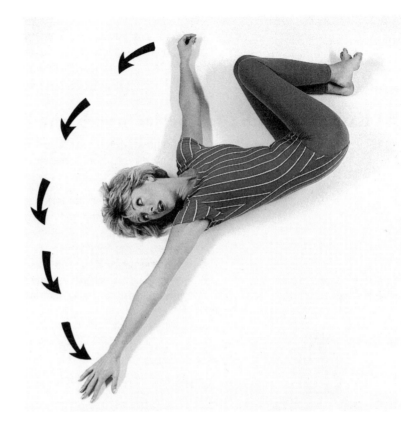

movement range has been fully reached and a little expanded. Too much stretching all at once can cause problems: the muscles get so angry they hurt and retract further than where you started. A little stretching every day will get you a lot further than violently stretching once a week.

Ⓘ Exercise No.81   Throwing Off Upper Back Tension

Standing strongly and evenly with your feet shoulder width apart, let your arms hang loose by your sides.

1. Throw your whole right arm with a strong and rapid movement over and across your left shoulder. The action should come from your right shoulder blade and at the end of the movement you should let go of any upper back and arm tension, leaving the action to momentum.
2. Repeat this throwing movement of the right arm eight times, and at the same time bend your head down to look over your left foot. This combination of posture and action will lengthen the muscles and release the tension in the right side of your upper back and shoulder.
3. Finish by shaking the arm loose. Repeat with your left arm, this time looking down to your right foot.

You might, during these swinging and throwing exercises, hear the occasional cracking of bones in your shoulder or in part of the upper spine and shoulderblades. As long as you don't work too quickly, there is no danger. Don't worry about cracking noises — they are only an indication that things are beginning to move again inside your body.

(A) Exercise No.82

Shoulder Stretch with Forward Bend

The shoulder stretch with forward bend works not only on the shoulder joints but also on short hamstrings and allows the neck muscles to relax downwards in the upside down position.

1. Stand firmly in a wide stride and interlock your fingers behind your back. Now turn your palms down towards your body so that they are facing backwards. This movement makes your arms rotate outwards from the shoulder joint.
2. Keep your arms locked in this position and, leading with your head, begin bending slowly downwards to the floor, pulling your arms upwards until you feel their weight help you go down even further.

Fig 65: *Shoulder turn out with forward bend*

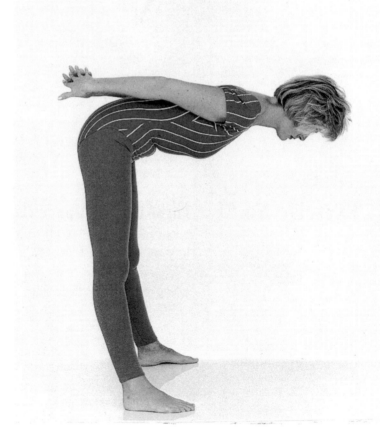

3. Stay hanging there for eight counts. Let your arms fall down towards the floor but keep your hands clasped together. Relax your neck and shake your head about.
4. If you spread your legs wider and go down far enough, your head and arms will eventually touch the ground.

(A) Exercise No.83   Back Hand Shake

Your body should be supple enough so that any of its parts can easily be touched by your hands. Imagine never having to ask someone to do your zip up or scratch your back!

Stand with your feet shoulder width apart and lift your right hand up over your right shoulder. Now try to shake hands with the left hand.

If your hands won't reach each other, hold a small towel or belt in your right hand, and grab the other end of the belt with your left hand, as close as possible to your right hand. With regular practice, your hands will soon be able to greet each other in this way. The back hand shake rotates your shoulder joints inwards.

Fig 66: *Back hand shake*

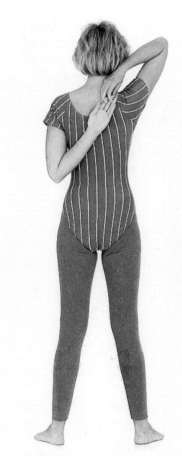

Ⓘ Exercise No.84 Arm Pulling

Pulling on a limb has a similar effect to hanging it by its extremity and it is an important aspect of keeping the body loose to allow free flow of electricity, lubricants and nutrients into the joints, tendons, muscles and skin.

1. Ask two good friends over for dinner one night and while waiting for the food to cook, ask them to stand by your sides, each at a distance equal to two arms' length away from you.
2. Now raise your arms up to shoulder height and ask your two friends to hold one of your hands each and pull. They must hold your wrists or fingers and lean away from you, pulling and shaking your arms away from the shoulder joint.

   The arm pulling exercise always makes people giggle. This is natural as giggling and laughing often go with release of tension.

Ⓑ Exercise No.85 Shoulder Shake on the Floor

An even better version of the arm pulling exercise is for you to lie flat on the floor rather than stand. The two friends should squat directly opposite your shoulders and watch each other to co-ordinate timing, or you will be shaken about like a rag doll. When you are up again from the shoulder shake you feel more alive. Do a few slow head rolls both ways to allow the energy you just gained to flow up into your head.

CHAPTER TWELVE

Your New Face

Ever since you started exercising, things have changed in your face. There are some little bits of your face which are only as old as the length of time you have been carrying out the exercise programme. Your chronological age is quite irrelevant: your skin, for example, renews itself fully every five years. This process slows down with age, but still the fact is that you are not now wearing the skin you were born with. The same applies to your hair and nails; for example, your big toenail is probably a couple of years old. It is not easy to accurately assess someone's true age in this way — let us say that some parts of our bodies are older than others. The fact that we were born on a certain date in history is merely one of many factors in our true age. Someone's talent in music, for example, may be as old as three centuries if that person comes from an ancient musical family.

Every time that an exercise is performed well and energy flows through your body, the area you are exercising is born again at that moment. This is exactly what happens in the Complete Facelift when it is properly carried out. But be careful: the Complete Facelift exercise which follows involves many other exercises combined. If you have not studied each individual section beforehand, you will not have learned the skills you need to perform this more advanced sequence, which involves almost every part of your face and head. You may try it if you wish, but the result will probably be a terrible mess at first, resulting in the most horrible grimaces. Please don't harm your face by being impatient! Only attempt to do the Complete Facelift when you are fluent at doing all the Beginners' and Intermediate exercises you have selected for your course. You will then only need to do a Complete Facelift as part of your everyday routine, plus a monthly half-hour booster session to remind you where everything goes or to deal with the most stubborn problem areas.

I do not recommend that you do a full facelift before going to sleep, as it will give you energy and wake you up. For bedtime practice, do a Full Facial Relaxation instead (page 42).

How Does it Work?

The Complete Facelift builds your face up starting from its base, at the clavicles. All the movements in the following sequence of short but intense massage, toning and relaxation routines are directed upwards from the neck to the crown. The power behind this exercise is that the action does not stop from beginning to end. For example, when you have massaged your neck and tightened the chin area to move on to your cheeks, you never fully let go of the parts that have already been toned, but keep them as a firm base for the following action. Although the Complete Facelift is not easy to do at first and quite demanding, it is most effective and takes no extra time at all. Once you can do it well, it need not take more than a few minutes a day, and can be carried out while you are washing, creaming, cleaning or feeding your face.

Ⓐ Exercise No. 86   Complete Facelift

Moisten your face, beginning at the clavicles and around the top of your shoulder blades, with a mild moisturiser: for example, tepid water and a little sweet almond oil and honey.

The complete facelift may be done in the upright, horizontal, or upside down positions (looking through the legs into a full-length mirror). A combination of all three, frequently changing planes, is more effective as this tones the face from all angles, attacking gravity on all fronts.

Each action described below should be performed to the following sequence of counts and breath:

A typical exercise wave

Count	1 2 3 4 5 6 7 8	1 2 3 4 5 6 7 8	1 2 3 4 5 6 7 8	1 2 3 4 5 6 7 8
Breathe	in		out	
Action	contract	hold	release	rest

1. Begin by massaging your neck starting at its base, where you can feel the clavicles, and at the back of the trapezius muscle (as far as you can reach down to your shoulder blades). Work your hands firmly upward from all directions. When you are working on the right side of your neck, bend your head to the left and massage with your left hand, and vice versa.

2. When you reach the area under your chin, stick your chin far up and out and stick your tongue out or press it firmly against the roof of your mouth. Feel the muscles under your chin getting tighter. Massage upwards and give 20 or more little taps on the contracted muscles

under your chin. This will firm them up even more.

3. Place the lip line and tone the mouth corners.
4. Smile a closed smile towards the earlobes.
5. Another, wider smile towards the cheekbones.
6. Perform a nose contraction without creating lines.
7. Keep the action flowing upwards, through the cheeks. Puff up your cheeks with air and gently tap them all over with the fingertips.
8. While keeping the rest of your face toned, massage the temples, ears and the back of the skull. Feel that your skin is loose and flexible, that it can move up over your bone structure.
9. Focus your eyes. Look up all the time from now on and concentrate on positive words or images ('It's a beautiful day today!' or you can no doubt think of your own examples). This instantly brightens your expression and really helps to keep everything in place all at once. Contract and release the lower eyelids, making sure no wrinkles are allowed to appear anywhere.
10. Expand the periphery putting emphasis on 1 o'clock and 11 o'clock.
11. Lift the eyebrows and the forehead to gather all your energy towards your scalp. Do upper lid contractions while holding your forehead and eyebrows high.
12. Massage your scalp, starting at the back of your neck and behind your ears, following the temporal muscle all the way up to your crown. Reach with the hands high up above your head, as far up as you can reach.
13. Now climb up high on to the balls of your feet and, still looking up, try to touch the ceiling.
14. Slowly lower your heels and arms, breathe and twist your thorax gently from side to side.
15. Find your lifted centre and you are ready to face a new day of vitality and alertness.
16. **But before you go.**.. check with an extra mirror held at right angles to your full-length mirror, where your head is in relation to your spine. Carry your new face in its proper centred position: chin down, back of the neck slightly retracted (pulled back) and your gaze just above the horizontal, with a pair of clear, open eyes.

Exercise No. 87

Upside down facelift

1. Stand with your back towards the mirror and your legs wide apart. Let your head drop towards the floor until you can see your face in the mirror through your legs.
2. Follow the same pattern of movements you have done in the previous exercise from 1 to 12. Work all the muscles in the face upwards towards your crown. Take your time over this and remember to breathe freely with the movements.
3. Slowly come back up to a standing position from the base of your spine, through the waist, ribcage, shoulders, neck and head in that order.

Carry on with Numbers 13 to 16 as in Exercise 86.

Exercise No.88

Horizontal Facelift

1. Lie on your back, flat on the floor.
2. Following the sequence of movements in Exercise 86, carry out Numbers 1 to 12, working each muscle in your face upwards towards the crown. When you finish No. 12, stay on the floor and stretch your arms, fingers, legs and toes as far out as they will go in a star shape to finish the sequence.
3. Feel your relaxed body stretched out on the floor and enjoy a minute or two of complete rest. This allows you to collect your thoughts for the day's activities lying ahead.
4. When you feel quite ready, slowly open your eyes, roll over on to your front and get up to continue with Nos. 13-16 as in Exercise 86.

Your New Face

The exercises in this book have attempted to build you up from scratch. We started at the feet rebalancing the body, and learned how to walk and move economically and gracefully. It is quite likely that you now have tried many if not all of the beginners' exercises in the book. It is hoped that your movement vocabulary is considerably expanded; that you spend more time in the horizontal and perhaps even in the upside down position. But first and foremost, your face should now be looking and feeling a lot better than it did when you started.

What are you going to do next? Is the book going to be tidied away on a bookshelf to gather dust next to the yoga book and all the other books you don't look at any more? No, I suggest you keep the book either in the bathroom, if you have a nice big bathroom with space for books and magazines, or alternatively, you could keep it in the kitchen with your cookery books. If you find a more detailed publication (see bibliography) on essential oils or aromatherapy, keep that in the same place, with the oils. You should have your exercise plan pinned up next to the bathroom mirror or dressing table, somewhere conveniently at hand, and do your daily exercises before even finishing your cleansing routine. In addition to this, you should remember which habitual facial expressions you have chosen to get rid of and try to stick to your newly learned practices throughout the day, in order to maintain good postural and facial habits.

Every morning when you wake up, face life afresh. If you did any exercises yesterday, some little bits of you are newly born today. Are Arnold Schwarzenegger's biceps as old as he is? No. Each newly developed piece of muscle is new, perhaps just a day old. When you get up in the morning your face might feel a little puffed up and tight, particularly if you have been exercising very hard. That is just the same as when your body feel sore after a hard workout. The pain is a mixture of acid left in the muscles, meaning you did not relax a muscle enough after exercise, plus newly developed little muscle units (babies, you could call them) making themselves known to you. The best remedy against muscle pain is to use the same muscles again. This will get rid of acidity and supple up the muscle. The pain goes as soon as you start moving, but you have to make an effort to start when you body feels unwilling.

It will be relatively easy for you to keep your face looking fresh, fit, happy and healthy from now on. You will remember that I promised you visible improvements in your looks by practising for 10 minutes a day for two weeks. Have you achieved any visible results? Have you been practising for 10 minutes a day?

If, after only such a short time of practice, you think that your face needs a lot more working on, you are probably right. Major improvements won't happen over a fortnight. How quickly you progress is now up to you. But before you do any more, take a whole week's rest from exercising and allow your body to get used to all the new messages you have been giving it. Towards the end of the week, that is if you have completed the introductory course, (10 minutes a day for two weeks) you may plan a new course (by means of the Exercise Charts in Chapter 3), and resume practice next week with intermediate or advanced exercises for three weeks (for 10 minutes daily) until you can follow the Complete Facelift at the beginning of this chapter. After that, provided you incorporate the Complete Facelift in your daily cleansing routine, you will only need to do the following in addition to the beginners, intermediate, advanced exercises that make up your courses.

- Daily:
  Ten minutes a day as part of your cleansing routine time. Do any amount of facial exercises while washing, in the bath or under a shower, while putting on make-up, brushing your hair or teeth etc.
- Weekly:
  Feed the face
  Have a deep cleansing massage or facial sauna
- Monthly:
  Half hour 'boosters'. Choose your favourite exercises, the ones that are the most effective for you. It is a good idea to change your routine monthly to discover new feelings in your face and to prevent the practice becoming boring. During these reassessment periods, look in the mirror and notice what parts of your face you are satisfied with and what parts need attention. You can then go back to the book, look up the part that needs attention and do something about it there and then. If, for any reason, you have been doing an exercise for a while and you find it does nothing for you at all, go back to the book and read the

instructions again slowly. You may have bypassed something vital. If the exercise still doesn't work for you, drop it. There are enough alternative exercises for each part of the face to give you a choice, and you may not want to use them all.

Be Prepared

It is a good idea to plan your life ahead and take good periods of rest and exercise when your face needs to be in top form. Then, shortly before an important date, be it romance, business, or a public appearance, you can treat yourself to some vigorous rejuvenating exercises that will not only make you look fit and alive, but also make you feel more confident to meet the challenges ahead. In the context of this book, the immediate challenge is to succeed in toning up your face with everlasting results. The only way you are going to achieve this is by practising the exercises. Never give up. To give up is the same as losing interest in yourself. And if you are not interested, then who else is going to be? You may take a break, forget about your face completely, but never for more than about a week; after that break, reinstate facial exercise as part of your daily routine.

The Body is Naturally Lazy

Now I have said a lot of nice things about the body in the course of this book, but one thing I must add here is that the body is naturally lazy. If you observe a domestic animal which is well-cared-for, it will be sleeping day and night. When it is stimulated to move, however, it seems as agile as an Olympic athlete. Why is this? Because the animal is relaxed fully unless action is called for. It does not waste physical energy being uncomfortable. It is allowed to stand, sit, lie, roll, jump — in short, its movement vocabulary is much wider than ours. We can be just as lazy as a dog or cat; the trouble is that a) lying down during the day is considered to be indulgent and b) we have to spend most of our waking hours exclusively in the upright position, dressed in tight clothes, sitting at hard, square furniture, surrounded by box-like buildings and fuming vehicles. So I come back to the key point of the book which is comfort. Ageing should not have to be accompanied with discomfort. **Discomfort is a sign of pain and shows externally as ugliness**.

It may seem that the present culture of the West is a role model for the rest of the world, but it appears from studying our own habits that we have not yet managed to create a truly comfortable environment for ourselves to live in. An overdose of useless consumer goods, products and services are pushed down our throats by mega-companies whose sole aim is to make money and more money. The long-term lack of clean air, horizons, sunsets, and so many other natural things that don't cost anything, may be just as damaging to our health as chain-smoking; who can tell? Knowledge from less 'civilized' cultures is so readily available to so many people in the Western world; these cultures act as mirrors to our own systems of values. Social values are, more often than not, merely the perpetuation of old habits. People are naturally conservative and, once settled, they don't like to change. Habit, however, the most cruel form of slavery, always forces us to maintain a *status quo* that is no longer relevant.

I hope that learning in this book about movement and expression in your face has taught you a little more about movement in general, and shown that the movements of each and every individual make up the movement character of their culture. For a culture that likes to call itself exemplary, we may safely rid ourselves from long-standing habits, born in the Middle Ages, that are no longer comfortable. The traditional female shape in the West stems from a centuries-old, tightly corsetted figure-of-eight shaped body with a wasp's waist and bulging bosom and hips. This evolved into the current traditional Barbie Doll with her long stork-like legs and high heels, ready to be pushed over at any time to be 'serviced' by macho Ken holding a gun in his hand. While we ponder introspectively over our individual facial features, we are learning how the body works, feels and responds, so in time we may begin to change the face of women and men in the West, to offer role models that we, as ordinary people, may feel more comfortable with.

A woman today does not have to lose her looks with age. With care, knowledge and practice, she can remain strong, healthy, happy, in one word, beautiful for the whole of her life.

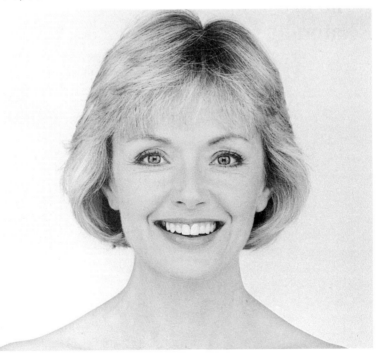

APPENDIX

List of Exercises

Ⓑ = Beginners
Ⓘ = Intermediate
Ⓐ = Advanced

Ⓑ 1 Feet Placement
Ⓑ 2 Pliés, Rises and Squats
Ⓑ 3 Pelvic placement (1)
Ⓑ 4 Pelvic placement (2)
Ⓑ 5 Waist Toners
Ⓑ 6 Ribcage Articulation
Ⓑ 7 Loose Arm Swings and Circles
Ⓑ 8 Shoulder Placement
Ⓑ 9 Neck Articulations
Ⓑ 10 Full Facial Relaxation
Ⓑ 11 Regeneration
Ⓑ 12 Upside Down Face
Ⓘ 13 Ironing Out Pressure Points
Ⓑ 14 Abolish Cellulite
Ⓐ 15 Underwater Neck Roll
Ⓐ 16 Cleaning the Nasal Passage
Ⓑ 17 Ear Popping
Ⓑ 18 Head Placement
Ⓘ 19 Scalp Knock
Ⓘ 20 Horizontal Head Butt
Ⓘ 21 Upright Head Butt
Ⓑ 22 Sideways Brushing
Ⓑ 23 Forward Brushing
Ⓑ 24 Backward Brushing
Ⓑ 25 Hair Shakes
Ⓑ 26 Circular Hair Shake
Ⓘ 27 Upside Down Hair Shake
Ⓐ 28 Figures of Eight
Ⓑ 29 Feeling the Temporal Muscles
Ⓑ 30 Ironing Out Wrinkles
Ⓘ 31 Rubbing Out Wrinkles
Ⓐ 32 Elimination of Worry Line
Ⓑ 33 Ironing Out a Frown
Ⓘ 34 Frown Stretcher
Ⓐ 35 Ironing the Forehead
Ⓑ 36 Relaxing the Eyes
Ⓑ 37 Eliminating Puffy Eyelids
Ⓑ 38 Eye Bag Removal
Ⓑ 39 Crow's Feet Extinction
Ⓑ 40 Expanding the Periphery
Ⓑ 41 Focusing
Ⓐ 42 Sun Focusing with Care
Ⓘ 43 Focusing in the Dark

All facial exercises in this book are a part of the Kando Technique devised by the Kando twins, Juliette and Madeleine. The Kando Technique (KT) is being taught at the Every Body studios. There are at the time of publication two Every Body studios, one in England and one in the U.S., with further outlets planned in Amsterdam, Berlin, Budapest and San Francisco. For more information please contact:-

EVERY BODY in Europe:
Juliette Kando
88 Victoria Road, London NW6 6QA, U.K.
tel (0171) 625 6577

EVERY BODY in the United States:
Madeleine Kando
4 Elmbrook Cricle, Bedford, Massachussets, U.S.A.
tel (617) 275 3690

BIBLIOGRAPHY

A Scented Well of Health: Etheric Oils, Rita Carpentier (Dekave, Alkmaar 1987)

The Vitamin Herb Guide: Natural Treatment for 150 Common Ailments, (Global Health Ltd., Alberta, Canada 1987)

Enchanting Smells, Suzanne Fisher-Rizzi (De Driehoek, Amsterdam,1988)

Soignez-Vous à la Chinoise, Dr G. Grigorieff (Marabout, Alleur, Belgium 1987)

Acupuncture, Dr Felix Mann (Pan Books, London 1985)

Acupressure Techniques, Dr Julian Kenyon (Thorsons, London 1987)

Soft Exercise, Arthur Balaskas and John Stirk (Unwin Paperbacks, London 1983)

Food Combining for Health, Doris Grant and Jean Joice (Thorsons, London 1984)

The Body in Question, Jonathan Miller (Jonathan Cape Ltd, London 1978)

Natural Facelift, M. J. Saffon (Arlington Books, London 1981)

Lindsay Wagner's New Beauty, Lindsay Wagner and Robert M. Klein (Piatkus, London 1988)

The Mechanical Foundations of Human Motion, J. V. Krause and Jerry N. Barnham (The C. V. Mosby Co., Saint Louis 1975)

The Aromatherapy Handbook: The Secret Healing Power of Essential Oils, Daniele Ryman (Century, London 1984)

Our Bodies, Ourselves, Boston Women's Health Collective, (Penguin Books, London 1989)

The Book of Yoga, Lucy Lidell (Ebury Press, 1983)

How to Grow and Use Herbs, Ann Bonar and Daphne MacCarthey (Ward Lock Ltd, London 1974)

Herbal Manual, Harold Ward (Fowler & Co. Ltd, London 1969)

Ageless Ageing, Leslie Kenton (Arrow Books, London 1985)

Better Eye Sight without Glasses, William Bates (Mayflower Books, 1979)

The Body as a Medium of Expression: Collection of Essays in Social Studies, (Penguin Books, London 1975)

The Whole Health Manual, Patrick Holford (Thorsons, London 1988)

INDEX